THE DIF...
between
PAIN and SUFFERING

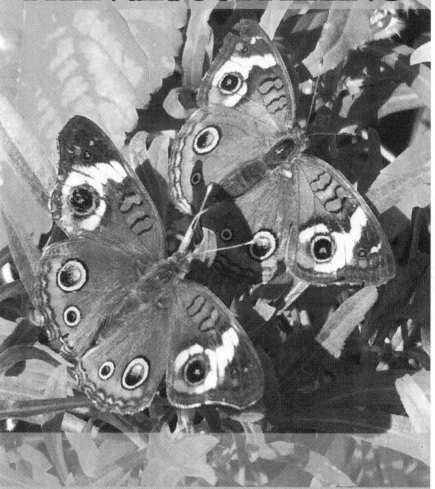

CATHERINE CARRIGAN

Book design by RamaJon
Bikeapelli Press, LLC

Cover Photo by Catherine Carrigan
Yoga photos by Diane Fulmer
Acupuncture pictures licensed from
www.123rf.com

Available for order through Ingram Press Catalogues
Catherine Carrigan

Visit my websites at
www.catherinecarrigan.com
www.unlimitedenergynow.com
www.whatissocialmediatoday.com

Printed in the United States of America
First Printing: August 2017

ISBN: 978-0-9894506-3-8

Table of Contents

~ 4 ~

Introduction: The Difference Between Feeling the Rain and Getting Wet

"Some people feel the rain, others just get wet."
- Roger Miller

One sunny afternoon in September 2013, I found myself semi-daydreaming on a long car trip.

Being a medical intuitive healer, I do most of my writing intuitively, waiting for guidance about what to write about. When I write, it feels as if I am simply taking dictation, also known as channeling.

My guidance that dusty late summer day was very clear: Write an article about the difference between pain and suffering.

When I finally got to my computer, it took less than half an hour. I didn't think much about what I wrote because the information seemed so obvious to me. Virtually every day of my life, I empower people to get out of pain and relieve suffering.

I didn't give the article another thought until several months later when I began noticing who was actually coming to www.catherinecarrigan.com and what they kept wanting to read.

Even four years later, somebody reads that article every single day.

I realized after watching the constant attention to this subject that I was being called for further explanation. So many people have been harming themselves in their quest for relief from pain and suffering.

In the U.S., opioid use has reached epidemic proportions. "Among 47,055 drug overdose deaths that occurred in 2014 in the United States, 28,647 (60.9%) involved an opioid," the Centers for Disease Control reports.

That means more people are dying from pain killers than car crashes.

Drug overdose is now the No. 1 cause of death for Americans under the age of 50.

Oxycontin and other hard-core prescription medications have become the leading gateway drugs to heroin. These harmful drugs set people up for long-lasting changes in their brains that cause depression and speed up cognitive decline.

This book, *The Difference Between Pain and Suffering*, is my humble attempt to summarize what I say to my clients -- advice that works based on my 24 years in natural healing.

My prayer goes from my soul to your soul that these words will transform not just your pain and suffering but your entire life.

May you experience radiant health, excellent vitality and a happy heart as a result of the words you begin to take in now.

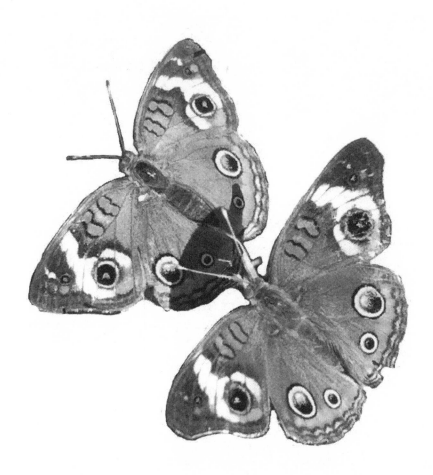

Book 1:

Your Pain Points

Chapter 1: The Difference Between Pain and Suffering

"Out of suffering have emerged the strongest souls; the most massive characters are seared with scars."
- Khalil Gibran

There's a difference between pain and suffering.

Pain is the physical experience. It's an ache in your muscles, the strain in your joints, the fever and chills, the throbbing in your temples, the congestion in your sinuses, the stabbing in your upper back, the shooting sharpness down your leg.

Suffering is your emotional experience. Suffering may or may not be connected to physical pain. You can suffer emotionally even on a sunny day when nothing apparently bad is happening to you on the outside. Suffering is the negative story you are telling yourself about what is happening now, what has happened in the past or what could potentially happen in the future.

I'm a medical intuitive healer.

That means -- in a nutshell -- that I use my intuition to read your body to figure out not only what's wrong but what will work to make you better.

During a medical intuitive reading, part of what I do is help you to understand:

- The physical causes of your pain and the natural healing approaches that will alleviate it.

- The emotional causes of your suffering and the spiritual healing approaches that will lift you out of your condition.

As human beings, sooner or later we experience the vicissitudes of life. The rain comes. We lose our job. The value of our investments goes down. We stub our toe, break our foot, catch a cold, contract an infection, or get a bad report from our doctor.

When these things happen, it's easy to take it all personally, as if somehow nobody other than you is going through anything half as challenging.

From a spiritual perspective, it's helpful to understand that pain is an aspect of our collective human experience. We all experience birth and death, two of the most traumatic events that will ever happen.

During a healing with a client, part of what I do is thresh out the difference between your physical pain and your emotional suffering.

It's my experience that if you try to get rid of a physical pain without also clearing the emotions behind the pain – the suffering – you won't be able to clear the pain totally. It may morph into another direction, another organ, another layer of your energy field.

So, if I am doing a healing, I identify the goal – say to get rid of your shoulder pain – and then find the emotion or emotions plural behind the pain. Once I identify all aspects of the story of your suffering about the physical pain, I lock the information into your subconscious mind and clear the whole thing – pain *and* suffering – at the same time.

Many people are unable to get rid of their pain completely because they haven't confronted themselves about their suffering.

We can be so heavily invested in our tales of sorrow and woe that we have no clue how much repeating that negative story creates the chemistry in our body mind that triggers the physical pain.

Next time you are in physical pain, pause to ask yourself, "What is the emotion I am suffering with this?"

Identify your emotions in as much detail as you can.

If possible, see if the feelings began at an early age in

your life. Many times our negative story started very early – even at birth. Sometimes we know this story because we have told it to ourselves so many times.

The quicker you can let go of your emotional suffering, the sooner you can be done with your physical pain.

Chapter 2. What Is Your Pain Body?

"We are what we are because we have been what we have been."
- Sigmund Freud

Simply put, your pain body is the same thing as your unresolved emotional baggage.

When you walk around with a backlog of pent-up feelings, the weight and density of that energy can literally short-circuit your entire mind-body system and shut down any other level of your being.

Don't believe me? Let me tell you a story.

In 2004 I was on vacation in Los Angeles. I was driving a rental car on my way to a yoga class in Santa Monica when my cell phone rang.

The person on the other end of the line delivered dreadful news: My beloved mentor from Brown University, Professor Kermit Champa, had just died.

Up until that point, I had spoken with him virtually every week for 24 years. He had been the father I always wanted but never had.

Suddenly he was gone.

Even though I was well-rested, well-fed and eager to practice yoga, when I arrived at the class, all I could do was lie on my mat. I could barely move.

The loss hadn't just brought me to tears. It had immobilized me.

For days, weeks and months afterward, I struggled to bring myself back into balance.

Perhaps you can recall a similar experience where a sudden, highly charged event changed literally everything about you.

Here's a simple way to understand why emotions can have such a profound effect:

- Your spiritual body controls your intellectual body.

- Your intellectual body controls your emotional body.

- Your emotional body controls your energy body.

- Your energy body controls your physical body.

Simply understanding this fact can save you years of pain and suffering.

To solve a problem on one level, you will want to reach up to the higher level for your solution. You can think of each of these bodies as levels of power:

- Your soul controls your mind. That's why, as we develop our spirituality, we can become mentally stronger and more capable of withstanding the vicissitudes of life. That is why many frail elderly people have become like spiritual warriors. Even though they may not be as physically strong as they used to be, they become great pillars for their entire community.

- Your mind controls your emotions. As you look for the wisdom rather than the hurt in all of life's challenges, you can save yourself enormous amounts of emotional pain. That's why thinking positively, looking on the bright side, having a sense of humor and reframing your challenges can soften the blows you feel emotionally.

- Your emotions control your energy. You can learn how to feel your feelings and let them go – as opposed to either running away from them through addictions like drugs (legal and illegal), alcohol, sex, overworking and the hundreds of other ways you can ignore what's really going on. A good way to think of emotions is that they are a process. As you develop healthy stress management skills, you can process through the inevitable hurts more easily. I often work with young teens and have tremendous compassion because they haven't yet learned how to handle all their emotions. They can easily be derailed by disappointment, divorce, death and the challenges of growing up. No matter what your age, the more you develop successful methods of handling your emotions, the healthier you will be in every way.

- Your energy body, which includes your chakras, your acupuncture meridians and your breath, controls your physical, material reality. That is why when your chi is depleted, you can feel so physically weak.

Your physical body is the densest part of who you are.

A good way to think of your physical body is that it is the result of your energy, your emotions, your mind and your soul.

By the time you experience pain and suffering, the causes have been with you for some time. That's because energy enters through your spiritual body, filters down into your mind, spreads to your emotions and then your energy body and finally materializes in your physical body.

If I am working with a client to relieve pain and suffering, we have to reverse the process. That means you must move the vibration of pain and suffering back out of your physical body, through your energy, through your emotions, through your mind and all the way past your spiritual self.

Simply put, pain comes in through your spiritual body, past the gateway of your mind, into your emotions where things can get quite tumultuous, through your energy and finally into your physical organs, glands, bones and muscles.

As a result, if you've been working to get rid of pain only through your physical body, you may not have been very successful.

To get rid of your pain and suffering, you must honor who you really are and take all five bodies into account.

Recently I was working with a new client who had been suffering from chronic low back pain. Although she had worked regularly with a chiropractor, a masseuse and a craniosacral therapist, improved her nutrition and started practicing yoga, nothing could get rid of the chronic, nagging ache on her right side.

She came to me for a medical intuitive reading.

Very quickly I explained that 30 percent of her pain was due to a low-functioning right kidney, 40 percent due to severe adrenal burnout and the last 30 percent due to spiritual loneliness. Her soul was longing for the companionship of like-minded people.

Even though she is happily married and has two well-behaved children and a fulfilling part-time job, she admitted she had been praying to find people she could really talk to. "If you think I'm tired now, you should have seen me years ago," she told me.

Her self-care and great attitude indeed made a difference but had not cleared her low back pain completely.

I explained the way energy flows in your body:

- Energy enters the crown of your head through the bahui point.

- The hara line is a vertical electrical current running through the bahui all the way down into the center of the earth. Any breaks, blowouts or disruptions in your hara line can lead to major disruptions in your energy flow.

- Your hara line feeds energy into your chakras. Your chakras are vortexes of energy located throughout your body. People who practice energy exercise such as yoga, tai chi and qi gong are doing themselves a wonderful favor by balancing these energy centers. Although these forms of exercise may be gentle, their benefits are profoundly beneficial. The more balanced your chakras, the more balanced your endocrine system and every organ system in your body will be. In addition to energy exercise, you can visit a highly trained energy healer such as myself to clean out and repair your chakras.

- Your chakras feed your acupuncture meridians. Your meridians are like rivers of energy. In addition to acupuncture, other forms of energy healing including acupressure, Reiki and hands-on healing. A block in your acupuncture meridians may be the cause of your pain.

- Your acupuncture meridians feed your organs. In my client's case, after all her chiropractic treatment, massage, craniosacral therapy, yoga and good nutrition, it was a surprise for her to hear that her right kidney and right adrenal gland had been contributing to her pain. Food healing, nutritional supplements, adequate hydration and energy work as well as yoga, tai chi and qi gong can all help rebuild the chi in your organs.

- Your organs feed your muscles. If you have chronic muscle pain, you can learn which organs are related to that muscle. The healthier your organs, the less muscle pain you will feel.

Your entire body is like one big hologram. Each aspect is deeply interrelated to other aspects of yourself. When you suffer pain, the more you inquire about the correlations between these different aspects, the more likely you are to root out the causes and resolve the issue.

Every organ carries emotions that may be adding to your pain body. For example, your large intestine acupuncture meridian relates to your colon. The muscles correlating with that meridian include the quadratus lumborum muscle in your lower back as well as your hamstrings. If you have low back pain, more than likely these muscles are highly involved in your suffering.

That is why if you came to me for corrective exercise and therapeutic yoga for low back pain, more than likely I would recommend exercises to lengthen your hamstrings and balance the two sides of your quadratus lumborum muscles.

The emotions associated with your large intestine include:

- Guilt
- Grief
- Regret
- Release
- Self-worth
- Enthusiasm
- Depression
- Letting go
- Indifference
- Mercy
- Compassion
- Sadness
- Apathy

Most of the time we believe the world outside of us is the cause of the emotions we feel.

As a long-time medical intuitive healer, I am here to tell you the truth: What you feel is inside of you.

If you feel angry, you will look out into the world and find things to feel angry, bitter and upset about. If you feel depressed, you will look out and find 100 reasons to feel sorrowful.

As you shift your inner experience, the world you experience also changes.

You cannot get rid of your pain unless and until you shift your emotions.

If I am doing a healing – no matter whether it's to get rid of your back pain, improve your business, get to the bottom of your money issues or mend the relationship with your mother – after setting the goal, the very next thing we would do is find the emotions that have prolonged your suffering.

Why is this so important? Simply put, you cannot get rid of your pain unless and until you have resolved the emotions that have held it in place.

If you don't resolve those emotions, you simply morph the energy from one part of the body to another.

You fix your hurt knee, then your wrist goes wonky.

You fix your knee and your wrist, and then your foot starts hurting.

And so on.

You can think of emotions like vibrational patterns. The lowest-vibration emotions include:

- Scorn
- Hate
- Craving
- Anxiety
- Regret
- Despair
- Blame
- Humiliation

All true healing must include emotional healing.

As you resolve these emotions in yourself, you stop emitting this vibrational pattern.

As you stop feeling these emotions, you stop lighting up the parts of your brain related to the corresponding acupuncture meridians.

As you clear this energy from all parts of your body, you'll start feeling lighter and less bothered by your pain. This is why integrated holistic healing is often the fastest, most efficient way to clear your pain for good.

This is why I, as a medical intuitive healer, work on all five bodies – your spiritual, intellectual, emotional, energetic and physical selves.

Let me share a personal story that illustrates what I'm talking about.

In the fall of 2015, I was practicing yoga when I noticed my left wrist was hurting. I had just come out of a deep back bend. Even though I had learned the correct form so as not to strain my wrist, I felt a sharp, shooting pang. As busy as I was, I didn't pay much attention until a few months later when I was practicing qi gong.

I lifted my left wrist and noticed a large protruding bump – a ganglion cyst.

It turns out that my mother also has a ganglion cyst, sometimes known as a Bible bump because an old-time remedy involved hitting it with a large heavy Bible to get rid of the bump. Her ganglion cyst is in the exact same place as mine, only hers isn't hurting any longer.

"I'm 58 years old and I can still blame something on my mommy," I joked with my yoga class.

Indeed, many of the vibrational patterns that cause our pain and suffering did not in fact start with us. These are called:

- **Genomes,** or genetic thought patterns.

- **Miasms,** or beliefs, habits and tribal thought patterns that we picked up from the culture we grew up in.

I identified the emotion behind my wrist pain (resentment) and began taking a flower essence to resolve the feelings.

Even if the pattern had started with my mother, it was now in my own cells. If I wanted to resolve the pain, I had to go all the way back to its source through my genome.

As I did so, I also received chiropractic adjustments as my carpal bones had become misaligned.

Eventually the pain lessened.

Then one day I noticed I had run out of the flower essence I had been taking to resolve the emotions behind my wrist pain. Thinking I might be over it by then, I didn't bother to start on my second bottle.

A few days after I ran out of the essence, I noticed my wrist pain had returned! I immediately began taking the second bottle and continued to process the emotions that had made me hurt so badly.

To get rid of pain and suffering from all levels of your being, you must take an integrated approach.

You can take an aspirin, call your chiropractor or visit your medical doctor for an X-ray or an MRI. I strongly support all these approaches and also can recommend many natural healing remedies for pain.

But when you really want to get rid of pain and suffering, you will want to ask yourself:

- Where did my pain start?

- What are the emotions I am feeling?

- How are my spiritual, intellectual, emotional, energetic and physical bodies involved in this pain?

By taking an integrated approach, you can supercharge your healing, resolve your emotions, shift the vibration and empty out your pain body.

What works to overcome pain and suffering? Healing happens when you honor who you really are and take advantage of this deeper knowledge to address all aspects of your being.

Chapter 3. What Is Your Light Body?

"Let your light so shine before men, that they may see your good works, and glorify your Father which is in heaven."
- Matthew 5:16

Just as you have a pain body that carries the heavy, uncomfortable energy of your suffering, you also have a light body.

What is your light body? Simply put, it is the radiance of your soul.

Holistic healing features numerous meditation techniques as well as energy-healing modalities designed to awaken the awareness of your light body. These techniques may suggest that you are somehow separated from your light body, and many of us do indeed forget who we really are. But the truth is you are a soul. As a result, you never really lose total touch with your light body.

The real you is always here. You just have to recognize the light within and give yourself permission to radiate from your soul -- not only for your own benefit but for the blessing of all others.

"Neither do men light a candle, and put it under a bushel, but on a candlestick; and it giveth light unto all that are in the house."
- Matthew 5:15

What if awakening your light body was as simple as seeing the light within yourself, ceasing your identification with your pain and suffering and appreciating the beautiful soul you really are?

What if you gave yourself permission to take such great care of yourself that you steadfastly resolve your core emotional conflicts and heal the diseases of your physical body?

You can be truly radiant, amplifying the glory of who you really are and becoming a source of inspiration to all others.

Your light can shine so brightly that you and other people can clearly perceive your magnificent soul.

Medieval artists depicted the halos of Jesus and the saints in countless images. These individuals became so identified with their spiritual bodies that their light illuminated all around them.

"Your vision will become clear only when you can look into your own heart. Who looks outside, dreams; who looks inside, awakes."
- Carl Jung

Often we see the agony of life as the only thing that's real. We feel inside ourselves and connect with the hurt, then look out into the world and project our hatred, judgment, division and troubles. At times, the agony can feel like the most real thing we have ever experienced.

Just the other day, I received a call for a medical intuitive reading from a lady suffering from trigeminal neuralgia, a disorder of the nerves in your face widely accepted in medical literature as one of the most agonizing conditions you can encounter.

"I've been suffering for two years and I don't think I can take it any longer," the dear lady said to me.

"I'm so sorry," I said to her with true understanding. Years ago I suffered from trigeminal neuralgia myself after a botched dental procedure.

At times of such intense agony, it can be easy to lose connection with your light body, but your light body is in fact who you are.

You are not your pain.

You are not your choices, either good or bad.

You are not your body, no matter how beautiful, healthy or strong it may be.

You are not your emotions, ebbing and flowing, going in and out like the tide.

You are your soul, a radiant body of light, eternal, of God, one with all that is, unbreakable, unstoppable, all-knowing, all-seeing, all-feeling, all-hearing and forever alive to your purpose.

Can you see it?

What works to overcome pain and suffering? Healing happens when you see your own light body and give yourself permission to shine that light for the benefit of all living beings.

Chapter 4. Where Does Pain Begin?
"The root of suffering is attachment."
- The Buddha

When you earnestly desire to feel better, a very smart question to ask yourself is: "Where did my pain begin?" To get to the root cause, it's important to understand how your body works -- not just your physical body but your *entire* self.

It's a law of physics that any vertical electrical current will have a magnetic field perpendicular to it. For humans, this magnetic field is called your energy field. Your whole body is electrical -- your heart can be measured through an electrocardiogram (EKG), and your brain waves can be measured through an electroencephalogram (EEG).

You may not think of yourself as an electrical being, but you emit energy all around you that can be sensed by both yourself and others.

In a nutshell, all disease, all pain, all suffering originates in this energy field and comes into your physical body.

By the time you feel discomfort, a disruption has been occurring in the flow of your personal chi for some time.

People who are extremely healthy and who have

developed their chi through practices such as meditation, yoga, tai chi, qi gong, healthy eating and adequate rest may have built an energy field that extends as wide as 100 feet in diameter.

For most of us, however, our energy field is much smaller -- more like eight feet in diameter.

You can think of this energy field as existing in layers even though in truth these layers overlap one another. Yogis, clairvoyants and other adepts have labeled these layers koshas.

Beginning in the outer layer, your spiritual body or Anandamaya kosha, literally translated as the body of bliss, controls your mind, or Vijnanamaya kosha.

From a practical perspective, that means when you experience pain, whether from a physical ache or a mental disturbance, the most powerful place to seek relief is at your soul level.

This explains why practices such as prayer, meditation and forgiveness can have such a profound effect alleviating your suffering on all levels.

Your mind controls your emotions, also called your Manamaya kosha. That's why when you change the stories you tell yourself and shift your inner dialogue from sorrow and woe to insight and understanding, you feel emotionally calmer and discover inner peace.

Your emotions control your energy body, also known as your Pranamaya kosha. You may have observed that when you feel happy, you experience unlimited energy, and when you feel rattled, upset, insecure, angry or fearful, the energy you have for living your life feels sharply diminished.

Your energy body controls your physical body, also known as your Anamaya kosha, which literally means the body of food. When your energy runs smoothly, you feel great physically.

When you understand that disease begins in your energy field -- literally out there in these layers -- you can begin a process of self-inquiry when you feel unwell.

What's going on spiritually?

What am I thinking?

What am I feeling?

How does my energy flow right now?
Is what I'm experiencing purely physical?

Even though it may appear that you just stubbed your toe, that you just went to the doctor and received an

unexpected cancer diagnosis, that you ripped the tendons in your right shoulder or you broke your leg in an accident, the truth is that somehow somewhere your energy field has been holding and grappling with this issue for some time.

As you begin to understand where your pain begins, you can take appropriate measures to find true relief. It's my experience that unless and until you identify the true source of your pain and suffering, the energy of that discomfort will simply shift from one area to the next.

You must address and resolve the actual issues.

As you find the courage to look at your whole being, you can discover and enjoy true relief at long last.

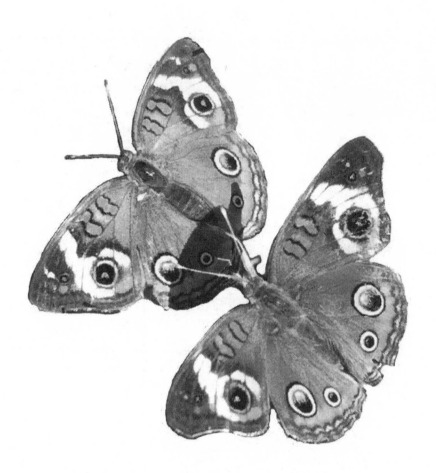

Book II.

Your Physical Body

Chapter 1. Is Your Pain Caused By What You're Eating?

"It is my impression that 'pain-killing' drugs improve the patient's mood rather than take away the pain."
- John E. Sarno

A client came to me complaining of skin rashes from head to toe. She felt so poorly she had made an emergency appointment with her medical doctor.

At the last minute, however, remembering she had reacted badly to medications for previous skin issues, she made an appointment to see me instead. I used kinesiology to determine (1) the root source of her problem and (2) what she could do to feel better immediately.

Even though she was not a heavy or even a regular drinker, she had downed a few too many alcoholic beverages on the previous Saturday night followed by an overdose of Halloween candy.

Through years of helping clients tackle all kinds of skin issues, I have found that the root cause is often a liver-kidney imbalance.

A lot of people understand that alcohol adversely affects your liver. Very few people know, however, that high-fructose corn syrup and sugar – the main ingredients in soft drinks and candy – are very similar to alcohol in that they must be metabolized by your liver.

As with alcohol, an overdose of candy, soft drinks and junk food can cause a fatty liver. In fact, there is even a name for it -- non-alcohol fatty liver disease.

A simple way to look at yourself to find out if you fall into this category is by checking if you have an extra roll of fat above your belly button. That would be your "liver roll" if you are unfortunate enough to have one.

Even if you don't drink more than 14 alcoholic beverages per week – the amount that technically would thrust you into the category of being an alcoholic – you may simply be eating more sweets than your liver can process.

High-fructose corn syrup is a common ingredient in not only soft drinks and candy but also cereals, breads, breakfast pastries, waffles, protein bars, ketchup, cookies, cakes, chocolate, yogurt, ice cream, jams, jellies, salad dressings, mayonnaise, corn chips, organic soups and BBQ sauce.

In other words, if you want to get high-fructose corn syrup out of your diet completely, you are going to have to read labels and think twice before eating any processed foods.

So back to my client with the head-to-toe skin rashes.

Her immune system was being suppressed, and she was reacting poorly to hand lotion, common painkillers and over-the-counter allergy remedies, organic coconut oil and more than 20 common foods she had been eating.

It was a good thing she had come to see a kinesiologist because I was able to ferret out which foods she could eat without getting a bad reaction. We further identified which kinds of lotion she could put on her body without aggravating the rash.

I encouraged her to use a far infrared sauna and take an oatmeal bath to calm her irritated skin. I gave her one supplement for detoxification and another to heal her gut and stop the bad reactions to multiple foods. I encouraged her to drink lots of distilled water to flush her kidneys.

A few days later, I saw her again.

"I feel so much better!" she told me. Not only had her skin improved, but her energy was better. Another, surprising side effect of cleaning the sugar out of her diet was that the aches in her joints had disappeared completely.

When you improve your eating and specifically avoid any foods that may be causing adverse reactions, your organs will be healthier and you'll have fewer if any muscle aches.

Your organs feed energy to your muscles.

You hold toxins in your joints.

If you take the time to detoxify, you will notice your joint pain going away.

Sometimes a bad reaction like a skin rash can be a blessing in disguise if we take the time to listen to our body.

Chapter 2. Nobody in Their Right Mind Eats CATS

"The basis of good health is always real, nutrient-dense food -- all other therapies depend first and foremost on the diet."
- Sally Fallon

Years ago, I was trying to come up with a simple, memorable way to explain to my clients how to eat smartly to get rid of their pain.

So here's my professional secret: Nobody in their right mind eats CATS.

Usually, if I explain this to you, your first impulse would be to laugh out loud. Laughing will help you to remember it.

If you have been truly suffering, more than likely you are willing to do whatever it takes to feel better.

Typically, you can cut your pain in half just by learning how to avoid inflammatory foods in your diet.

You can think of inflammation like fire in your body. It breaks down your hair, bones, muscle tissue and brain chemistry. It is a primary risk factor for cancer and a contributing factor for obesity.

If you have pain anywhere, you have inflammation, and you'll want to decrease your inflammation to get out of pain. It's that simple!

You do this by avoiding CATS and their unhelpful friends.

So what are CATS?

- Caffeine

- Alcohol

- Tobacco

- Sugar

CATS increase the levels of inflammation in your body. What are the friends of CATS?

- Fried foods

- Gluten

The friends of CATS are also highly inflammatory.

Now if you know anything about actual cats, you know they have a mind of their own. They cannot and will not be controlled. If you put them out, they want to come in.

If you keep them in, they want to go out.

Cats are the "crazy makers" of the pet world (yes, they are cute and fluffy, I'll admit).

If you think you have any control whatsoever over cats, you're wrong.

And so it is with caffeine, alcohol, tobacco, sugar and their unhelpful friends fried foods and gluten – not only the most pain-inducing habits on the planet next to bashing your head against the sidewalk but also the food groups you are least likely going to be able to control if you fool around with them regularly.

CATS and their friends are highly addictive. If you play with them long enough, they can take charge of your life, just like their furry four-legged cousins who sit on the dining room table, shed cat hair on your favorite jacket and give you a dirty look if you ask them to do anything other than what they want to do.

CATS can take such hold of your psyche you may believe you could never give them up:

- Forgo morning coffee?

- Reduce or eliminate beer, wine, mixed drinks?

- Give up cigarettes, cigarillos, cigars, chewing tobacco?

- Cut out sugar, candy, soft drinks, high-fructose corn syrup?

- Eliminate major food groups like fried foods, French fries, fried chicken?

- And get off gluten? Aside from the fact that it's been sprayed with glyphosate, which causes cancer, infertility, multiple sclerosis, autism, heart disease, gastrointestinal distress, obesity, depression and Alzheimer's, you may be totally hooked on your morning toast, cookies, cakes and pies.

But then one day you wake up in so much agony you can hardly stand yourself.

You are on every legal drug your doctor can prescribe and have tried all the ones from the drugstore, too.

Nevertheless, you can hardly walk around the block, raise your arm, bend over at the waist to tie your shoes or lift your finger without wondering what the hell happened to you.

Is it really worth allowing the CATS and their undermining friends to rule your life?

You can look up the inflammatory effects of any food by visiting www.inflammationfactor.com. This site uses a proprietary algorithm quantifying 20 different factors to explain the connection between what you put in your mouth and the pain you feel.

Whether a food raises or decreases your level of inflammation has to do with its amount and type of fat, its levels of vitamins, minerals and antioxidants, where it stands on the glycemic index and whether it contains anti-inflammatory compounds.

Foods with a negative number on the Inflammation Index are PRO-inflamatory and make you hurt more, including:

- French fries -51

- Fruit cocktail in heavy syrup -49

Foods with a positive number on the Inflammation Index are ANTI-inflammatory and make you hurt less, including:

- Acerola cherries +342

- Asparagus, cooked +38

When you make the effort to eliminate CATS and their misery-causing friends fried foods and gluten, you discover how much better you feel even without over-the-counter or prescription painkillers or non-steroidal anti-inflammatory drugs (NSAIDs).

Side effects of NSAIDs include:

- Stomach problems, including bleeding, ulcers and stomach upset

- High blood pressure

- Fluid retention

- Kidney problems

- Heart problems

- Rashes

Some people have so many other health issues that even their doctors advise against painkillers. People who need to consult their physicians before taking painkilling drugs include:

- Anyone with decreased kidney or liver function

- Patients with Crohn's disease or colitis

- Ulcer and gastritis sufferers

- Asthma patients

- Gastroesophageal reflux disease (GERD), acid reflux and hiatal hernia patients

- Anyone allergic to aspirin, other NSAIDs

- People taking blood thinners

- Pregnant women

- Anyone who drinks more than seven alcoholic beverages per week or more than two per day

- People over the age of 65

What works to overcome pain and suffering? Stop allowing CATS to rule your life.

Chapter 3. Juices and Smoothies Make Your Whole Body Smile

"There can only be one solution to any problem: a change in attitude and in consciousness."
- Greg Braden

Juicing is A-plus health behavior. Although many will hear about juicing, the few who are actually willing to do it get to enjoy:

1. Increased energy

2. Decreased food cravings

3. Gorgeous skin

4. The many benefits of live enzymes

5. Better digestion

6. Detoxification

7. Lowered cholesterol

8. Reduced inflammation

9. Weight loss

10. Natural healing for pain and suffering

If you decide to juice, talk yourself into making your own. Your cells will be so happy to receive food with the highest amount of life energy available!

There are many fancy juicers on the market. I recommend the Breville 800JEXL Juice Fountain Elite 1000-Watt Juice Extractor. My very first juicer was a Jack Lalanne Power Juicer. I went through several versions, replacing one after another when the motor would run out.

Health nuts will argue which is healthier: juices vs. smoothies. The truth is that smoothies win the health-nut battle due to the phytonutrients found in the seeds, peels and fiber of fruits and vegetables.

For smoothie making, I recommend a Blendtec Total Blender with the Wildside Jar, but many folks worship their Vitamix.

If you are new to juicing or smoothie making, I recommend you start with what I refer to as a "beginner juice" – carrots, celery and apple, or celery, cucumber and apple, or orange, ginger, lemon and carrot.

Another great juice that just about everyone enjoys is fresh organic lemonade. Buy a bag of organic lemons at your local health food store. Wash them and cut off the ends, but be sure to leave on the peels - the pectin they provide is great for your liver.

Run the lemons through your juicer and save the juice in a large jar. When you are ready for fresh lemonade, take one to two ounces of lemon juice, add the natural sweetener stevia to taste and fill the rest of your glass with filtered or sparkling water. Voila! The best lemonade you have ever tasted.

There are many recipes and books about juicing, but in my view, the general thought is simple: Half your glass should taste good. The other half should be good for you.

So, for example, half your glass could be fresh organic apple, pear or pineapple juice. The fruit juice will cover up the taste of the sharper vegetables like spinach and kale.

My favorite juice is spinach and apple along with parsley and Swiss chard I raise in my garden. Simply juice an entire box of organic spinach that you can buy at the grocery, then add an equivalent amount of Swiss chard and parsley. Finish it up with apples.

One of my favorite breakfasts is organic turkey sausages with a glass of fresh celery, parsley and apple juice.

Although I had heard of the many benefits of juices and

smoothies, what convinced me to start making them myself was meeting a neighbor. While out walking one day, I met this rosy-cheeked gentleman in his mid-90s.

He had a big smile on his face. I struck up a conversation and asked him to share his health secret.

"Juicing," he said.

"What do you juice?" I asked.

"Whatever is in the refrigerator," he replied.

You can see for yourself what happens at the cellular level when you start juicing.

A simple way to examine your health is to prick your finger, put a drop of blood on a slide and look at it under a microscope. You can see your cells and what is happening. When you don't get enough fresh fruits and vegetables, you can see fat globules floating around in your blood and the cell walls will appear squiggly.

I had done live blood cell analysis for years, but when I started juicing, the lady who examined my blood told me, "You have the healthiest blood of anyone I have ever seen!"

You can only look as good on the outside as your cells

are truly healthy on the inside.

Juicing can help you lose weight because your body will finally be getting the nutrients it craves. You will feel deeply satisfied and less hungry because you are finally giving your body the five to seven servings of fruits and vegetables it needs to function at its best.

Some common ailments and their helpful fruit and vegetable juices:

Acidity

Grapes, orange, cucumbers, carrot, kale, celery, pears, lemon, watermelon and spinach.

Acne

Grapes, pear, plum, tomato, cucumber, celery, carrot, pineapple, potato, broccoli, Swiss chard and spinach.

Allergies

Apricot, grapes, broccoli, carrot, kiwi fruit, garlic, beet, oranges, lemons and spinach.

Arteriosclerosis

Grapefruit, pineapple, pomegranate seeds, lemon, celery, goji berries, beets, strawberries, cucumber, lettuce, okra, cilantro and spinach.

Arthritis

Cherry, pineapple, sour apple, lemon, grapefruit, ginger, cilantro, papaya, turmeric, cucumber, beet, carrots, pineapple, lettuce and spinach.

Asthma

Apricot, lemon, pineapple, peach, kiwi fruit, carrot, strawberries, mango, cordyceps, mint, ginger, corn, dandelion root, radish and celery.

Bronchitis

Apricot, lemon, orange, pineapple, peach, tomato, garlic, papaya, red bell peppers, Swiss chard, collard greens, brussels sprouts, carrot, onion and spinach.

Bladder Ailments

Apple, apricot, lemon, cucumber, carrot, celery, parsley, radish, fennel, asparagus, cranberries, watermelon, grapefruit, lemongrass and watercress.

Cancer

Kale, spinach, garlic, celery, apple, beets, lemon, limes, papaya, garlic, cauliflower, Brussels sprouts, broccoli, beets, beet greens, berries, asparagus, oranges, ginger, avocado seeds, cayenne pepper and turmeric.

Colds

Lemon, orange, grapefruit, pineapple, carrot, onion, kale, garlic, celery and spinach.

Constipation

Apple, pear, grapes, lemon, carrot, beet, spinach, mint, avocado, guava, fennel, ginger, wheatgrass and watercress.

Colitis

Apple, apricot, peach, pear, pineapple, papaya, carrot, beet, cucumber, ginger, turmeric and spinach.

Diabetes

Citrus fruits, Swiss chard, berries, carrot, celery, lettuce, green apples, cinnamon, bitter melon and spinach.

Diarrhea

Papaya, lemon, pineapple, carrot, ginger, cranberries, fennel, spinach, beet greens and celery.

Eczema

Red grapes, carrot, apple, spinach, cucumber, cranberry, ginger, asparagus, watermelon and beet.

Eye disorders

Apricot, blueberries, tomato, carrot, goji berries, celery, bell pepper, lime, beet, apple, corn, parsley and spinach.

Gout

Red sour cherries, pineapple, tomato, turmeric, lemon, limes, pineapple, cucumber, beet, carrot, celery and spinach.

Headache

Grapes, lemon, carrot, lettuce, ginger, turmeric, Himalayan pink salt, Celtic sea salt and spinach.

Heart Disease

Red grapes, lemon, cucumber, celery, kale, carrot, beets, grapefruit, cayenne pepper, okra, beet greens and spinach.

High Blood Pressure

Grapes, orange, cucumber, celery, carrot, berries and beet.

Influenza

Apricot, orange, lemon, grapefruit, pineapple, ginger, garlic, carrot, onion, kale, thyme and spinach.

Insomnia

Apple, cherries, grapes, pears, Swiss chard, lemon, lettuce, carrot and celery.

Kidney Disorders

Apple, orange, lemon, cucumber, carrot, celery, asparagus, watermelon, cranberries, watercress, parsley and beet.

Liver Ailments

Lemon, apples, papaya, grapes, carrot, tomato, beet, parsley, beet greens, dandelion root and cucumber.

Menstrual Pain

Grapes, prunes, cherry, spinach, lettuce, ginger, turmeric, turnips and beet.

Prostate Troubles

All fruit juices in season, carrot, asparagus, lettuce, papaya, spinach and watermelon.

Rheumatism

Grapes, cherries, orange, lemon, grapefruit, tomato, cucumber, beet, carrot and spinach.

Sinusit

Apricot, lemon, orange, apple, tomato, carrot, kiwi fruit, onion, garlic, ginger and horseradish.

Skin Problems

Celery, cucumber, watermelon, cantaloupe, spinach, tomato, kale, parsley, strawberries, broccoli, radishes and grapefruit.

Sore Throat

Apricot, grapes, lemon, pineapple, prune, tomato, carrot, ginger, cayenne pepper and celery.

Stomach Ulcers

Apricot, grapes, pineapple, cayenne pepper, cabbage, lemon, wheatgrass, fennel, turmeric and carrot.

Tonsillitis

Apricot, lemon, orange, grapefruit, pineapple, carrot, spinach and radish.

Whether you create juices or smoothies, you reduce acidity that causes pain, increase your antioxidant reserves and set yourself up for speedy healing.

Chapter 4. Natural Healing Remedy for Pain

"Effective therapies treat the whole body as a unit."
-Pete Egoscue

You can easily make a drug-free, natural healing remedy for pain. In a juicer, put:

Ginger root

Small handful of turmeric root

One organic lemon

One golden beet

About 4-5 oranges, peeled

Why this recipe helps:

1. Ginger contains powerful, natural anti-inflammatory compounds called gingerols that suppress pro-inflammatory compounds cytokines and chemokines. Several scientific studies have proven that ginger relieves pain. In addition, a common side effect of many conventional prescription pain medications is nausea and vomiting. Ginger calms the digestive system and alleviates nausea. As little as one-fourth inch may provide relief. However, I usually throw in at least three inches of ginger when I am juicing for two people.

2. Turmeric is the yellow spice that gives Indian food its distinctive color. The volatile oil in turmeric is anti-inflammatory. The yellow pigment curcumin has been proven to be equally effective as the conventional pain medications hydrocortisone and phenylbutazone as well as over-the-counter medications but without the side effects.

3. Lemons are high in Vitamin C and also have antibiotic effects. When you go to the hospital, it's important to build up your immune system before and afterward. Lemons also have been proven to be an effective anti-inflammatory remedy.

4. Although red beets are beneficial, I like to use golden beets in this recipe. Turns out, you can sneak in healthier vegetables without anybody in your family noticing! Beets are anti-inflammatory because of their betanin, isobetanin and vulgaxanthin (say that real fast and I will give you a nickel!). In addition, beets are a good source of betaine, which regulates the inflammatory markers C-reactive protein, interleukin-6 and tumor necrosis factor alpha.

5. Oranges are high in Vitamin C to help you rebuild your immune system. The carotenoids in oranges (zeaxanthin and beta-cryptoxanthin) are also anti-inflammatory.

Why would you want to turn to natural healing to reduce your reliance on prescription medications?

Common side effects of heavy-duty pain medications include:

- Nausea or vomiting

- Skin rashes

- Liver damage

- Stomach upset

- Heartburn

- Kidney problems

- Fatigue and drowsiness

- Headaches

- Dizziness

- Swelling of the hands and feet

- Confusion and inability to think straight

You can look up the side effects of individual drugs, but I also recommend you examine how all your medications interact. More than half of Americans take more than one prescription drug.

You may have seen one doctor for one ailment and another physician for something else, and your medical team may not know how all your drugs interact.

By juicing regularly, you may be able to reduce or eliminate your reliance on prescription or over-the-counter pain relievers. Meanwhile, you will find yourself aching less, enjoying better energy, thinking more clearly and renewing your enthusiasm for healthy exercise.

You also can include ginger and turmeric throughout your diet.

It's easy to make ginger tea. Just wash fresh ginger root, slice it up and pour boiling water over it. Or allow your ginger tea to soak over time in a crockpot and drink throughout the day.

Chapter 5. Get Your Head On Straight to Relieve Pain

"The study of asana is not about mastering posture. It's about using posture to understand and transform yourself."
- B.K.S. Iyengar

Recently I worked with a new client who had been suffering from neck pain for some time. As an author, she spends many hours hunched over a computer.

Like many folks with desk jobs, she had not made the connection between the way she had been habitually sitting and the short, sharp shooting pains radiating from her neck into her left hand.

It wasn't that she didn't want to get better. In fact, she had undergone some 20 physical therapy sessions. But despite all her therapeutic efforts, the issue had not been resolved. She arrived at my office in a high degree of discomfort.

I started by measuring the exaggerated curvature of her upper back. Her thoracic spine measured 45 degrees, technically equaling kyphosis – a condition marked by a rounded upper back, a.k.a. hunchback.

The curve in your upper back ideally should equal no

more than 30 to 35 degrees. The greater your schlump, the worse your neck, shoulder and upper back pain.

Because my patient's upper back was so rounded, her head was jutting forward about seven inches in front of her shoulders. Every inch forward your head is leaning adds 10 pounds of pressure onto your neck. My patient looked like she was leaning into the heavy winds of life.

"You don't have your head on straight," I advised her.

"It's official."

Then I showed her how to sit properly in a chair. You can learn how to do this yourself by reviewing the exercises in the appendix of this book.

After my patient learned how to sit with good posture, her upper back straightened naturally and she could breathe more easily.

After I had positioned her in a chair, I asked, "How's your neck pain now?"

"Gone!" she replied, somewhat astonished, looking around as if she couldn't quite figure out what had happened. We had not done a single neck exercise.

Then I showed her how to stand properly.

I put a yoga block between her feet and another block between her inner groins and then had her lift the pit of her abdomen up toward the crown of her head.

Just by engaging her inner groins and pelvic floor, she could straighten her upper back. She breathed a quiet sigh of relief.

"Any pain now?" I asked.

Once again, no pain.

"This should show you that if you have shooting pain into your neck or hand, you aren't sitting or standing properly," I said.

I asked her to sit and stand again with no yoga props so she would know how to sit and stand anytime, anywhere, without discomfort. And then and only then did I begin teaching her the exercises to heal her neck.

If you've been working hard to relieve your neck pain, ask yourself if the problem isn't actually your upper back. Yes, the vertebrae in your neck may be out of alignment in any number of possible ways, but you will still have no hope of relief as long as your head is jutting out in front of you.

In fact, because the position of any joint depends on

good posture in the rest of your body, the pain you feel can probably be reduced when you learn good posture.

Your feet control your hips. Therefore, if you have achiness in your hips, you need to learn where to place your feet.

Your hips control your knees. If your knees hurt, you will need to balance your hips.

Your legs extend your spine. If your back hurts, you can reposition your legs.

The definition of good posture is the place where your body is most mechanically efficient. You may be astonished to learn how quickly you can rediscover comfort and ease when your body lines up properly.

When my client's session ended, her upper-back curvature was totally normal – 30 degrees. I had literally taught her how to put her head on straight.

Sometimes when we experience discomfort, we need to look at the larger picture of how our whole body is working together.

Get your head on straight, literally and figuratively! As you bring your body into alignment, your energy flows and your pain slows.

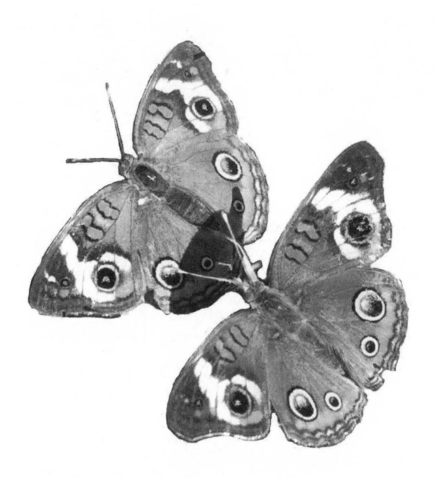

Book III.

Your Energy Body

Chapter 1. The Problem You Think Is the Problem Isn't Actually the Problem

"As a person thinks, feels and believes, so is the condition of his or her mind, body and circumstances."
- Joseph Murphy

When you look for true, long-lasting relief, you want to rid yourself of pain and suffering at its origin.

You've now learned there's a flow of energy in your body.

Energy enters your body through your hara line.

Your hara line is a vertical electrical current extending from above the crown of your head through the center of your physical body down into the earth.

Your hara line feeds prana into your chakras. Many people are familiar with the seven major vortexes called chakras, but you have minor chakras all over your body as well as above and below your body. Practices such as yoga, tai chi, qi gong, Reiki, energy healing and breath work can alleviate your suffering by restoring balance to your chakras.

Your chakras feed chi in to your acupuncture meridians. Many people have visited an acupuncturist or taken advantage of acupressure.

Your acupuncture meridians feed chi into your organs.

Your organs feed prana into your muscles.

As you study and come to understand this flow of energy in your body, you can begin to inquire within yourself if the problem is really your tight hamstrings or perhaps your large intestine that directs energy into your hamstring muscles.

Or whether the problem is really your large intestine or your large intestine acupuncture meridian or your first chakra or your hara line.

Where in fact do you experience energy leaks, too much or too little energy in your meridians, blockages, blowouts or shutdowns in your chakras?

You can take better care of your personal energy if you learn how.

Self-care practices such as yoga, tai chi and qi gong can restore balance to this flow of your personal prana and provide dramatic and often immediate relief.

Visiting an energy healer or acupuncturist can wipe away years of suffering.

Food healing such as juicing and smoothies, which give your cells the phytochemicals necessary to reduce inflammation and rebuild your organs, can alleviate systemic pain all over your body.

It's important to understand that just because you sense pain in one area of your body doesn't mean the disruption started in that location. More than likely, the pain didn't start where you actually feel it.

The more you see your body the way I do -- as a body of life energy that can be rebuilt in the same way you can save money and restore your savings account -- the more you will see how much hope you have for finding the ease and comfort you desire.

In fact, your personal energy is so crucial that the very first thing I do when I'm performing a medical intuitive reading is to examine your overall chi level. I measure your life energy on a scale of 0-to-100, with 50 being average for a man or woman of your exact same age.

People who have spent years focusing on excellent self-care often build their chi into the high 80s or low 90s.

Because we all face assaults from stress, toxic environments, inadequate rest, improper nutrition and not enough time for exercise, I rarely see anyone whose overall life energy is higher than the mid-80s.

On the other end of the scale, many people have neglected their personal health for so long that they pay attention when a doctor discovers a serious illness.

I like to think of life energy just like money: You have to spend it every day of your life, but you can also save, build and restore it.

You can heed the advice of wellness coaches, nutritionists, yoga, qi gong and tai chi teachers, psychologists and energy healers just like you can follow a savvy investment adviser.

As our health fails, our personal chi may drop into the 20s. When people are dying, their personal prana drops into the 20s and below.

We have to remember, however, that our health doesn't depend on our chronological age. You can be happy and healthy and enjoy excellent energy until the day you die - provided you take care of your personal chi.

Just like you can learn to manage your money wisely, you can learn how to maintain high levels of energy that feed every organ, muscle and cell and keep you pain-free until the day you die.

Chapter 2. Hidden Secrets of Your Chakras

"The spirit is the life of the body seen from within, and
the body the outward manifestation of the life of the
spirit -- the two being really one."
- Carl Jung

You can relieve pain and suffering by learning to take
better care of your chakras.

What are your chakras?

As we've discussed, your chakras are energy vortexes,
both large and small, located throughout your body as
well as your energy field. They are part of your
Pranamaya kosha, or energy body, and regulate the well-
being of your physical body as well as the quality of vital
energy you experience on a daily basis.

You're probably aware that it's a good idea to exercise
regularly, eat right, sleep well and manage your stress.

But who has ever told you that it's also a good idea to
balance your chakras?

And why is this a really good idea anyway?

Your chakras regulate the well-being of not only your
physical body but also your psychological experience.

When you experience physical pain or mental suffering, there's a 110 percent likelihood that a chakra corresponding to the area in your body or your emotional process has been out of balance for some time.

When I do a medical intuitive reading, I look at:

1. Your primary operating chakra, which tells me the filter through which you experience life.

2. The chakra or chakras that are out of balance.

Here is a simple guide to the hidden secrets of your seven major chakras. (You have other chakras throughout your body -- for example in your hands, feet and knees -- as well as below into the center of the earth and above the crown of your head.)

1st Chakra, Muladhara, Root Chakra

Location: Between your urethra and anus

Purpose: Our foundation

Issues associated with 1st chakra:

- Roots
- Grounding
- Trust

- Health
- Home
- Family
- Appropriate boundaries
- Prosperity
- Courage
- Vitality
- Self-confidence
- Survival
- Money
- Seat of kundalini

Signs you have a problem with your 1st chakra:

- Major illness or injury
- Disconnection from the body
- Fretful, anxious, can't settle down
- Poor focus, poor discipline
- Financial problems
- Poor boundaries
- Chronic disorganization

If your 1st chakra is excessive, you may experience:

- Hoarding
- Overeating

- Greed
- Fear of change, addiction to security
- Rigid boundaries

Color: Red

Glands: Adrenals

Developmental age:
2nd trimester in the womb to 12 months

Balanced characteristics:

- Good health
- Vitality
- Well-grounded
- Comfortable in your body
- Sense of trust in the world
- Feeling safe and secure
- Able to relax and be still
- Stable
- Prosperous
- Right livelihood

Physical malfunctions:

- Disorders of the bowel, anus, digestive system
- Adrenal burnout
- Disorders of the solid parts of the body: bones, teeth
- Issues with feet, legs, knees, base of spine, buttocks, hips
- Eating disorders
- Frequent illness
- Obesity

Affirmations that support your 1st chakra:

- I have a right to be here
- I am safe
- I love my body and trust its wisdom
- I live a life of abundance
- I choose to be here in this body in this lifetime
- I love my life
- I am meaningfully connected to my family
- I draw on my family for love and support
- I honor my connections to my tribe and transcend them
- I have plenty of money now
- I nurture my connection with nature

To heal wounds of your 1st chakra:

- Get hugged or held
- Create good bedding so you feel safe and comfortable as you sleep
- Garden
- Cook
- Take a walk
- Go barefoot
- Have a picnic
- Physical exercise
- Lots of touch, massage
- Reconnect with your body
- Look at your earliest childhood relationship to your mother
- Eat meat, proteins, red fruits and red vegetables
- Resolve old family conflicts
- Get out of survival mode and feel prosperous

Sound: Lam, C note

Yoga postures that benefit your 1st chakra:

- Standing poses, especially warrior poses, frog, butterfly, pelvic lifts, bridge, knee to chest, head to knee, seated boat, tortoise, eagle, lotus

2nd Chakra, Svadisthana, Navel Chakra

Location: Below your navel

Purpose: Balanced power and sexuality

Issues associated with 2nd chakra:

- Sexuality
- Ability to experience pleasure
- Power
- Creativity
- Intimate relationships
- Desire
- Sexual identity

If the 2nd chakra is deficient:

- Rigid physical body and attitudes
- Fear of sex
- Poor social skills
- Denial of pleasure
- Excessive boundaries
- Lack of desire, passion or excitement
- Powerless

If the 2nd chakra is excessive:

- Addiction to sex, drugs or alcohol
- Mood swings
- Excessive sensitivity
- Overpowering, invasion of others
- Emotional codependency
- Obsessive attachments

Color: Orange

Glands: Ovaries, testes

Developmental age: 6 to 24 months

Balanced characteristics:

- Graceful movement
- Emotional intelligence
- In your own power
- Comfortable with your own sexuality
- Able to change
- Healthy boundaries
- Emotionally balanced
- Ability to nurture self and others
- Ability to experience pleasure in healthy ways

Physical malfunctions:

- Disorders of the reproductive system
- Menstrual problems
- Sexual dysfunction
- Low back pain, knee trouble
- Lack of flexibility, either physically or emotionally
- Inappropriate appetite (either too much or not enough)

Affirmations

- I have a right to enjoy pleasure
- I accept and celebrate my sexuality
- I deserve to have fun
- I feel comfortable as a man/woman
- My sexuality is sacred
- My life is pleasurable
- I am flexible and go with the flow in life
- I nurture and support all my relationships
- I let go of all past emotional traumas
- I am creative

To heal wounds of your 2nd chakra:

- Give or receive massage
- Take a bath
- Work with your hands
- Swim
- Sit in a rocking chair
- Clean your house
- Feel music
- Inner child work
- Allow your hips to sway when walking
- 12-step programs for addictions
- Develop a healthy hobby just for fun
- Develop healthy boundaries
- Learn how to have healthy intimate relationships
- Honor your femininity/masculinity
- Eat orange fruits and vegetables

Sound: Vam, D note

Yoga postures that benefit your 2nd chakra:

- Forward bends, cobra, sphinx, boat, locust, bow, butterfly, child with knees apart, hip circles, pelvic lifts, hero, spinal twist

3rd Chakra, Manipura, Solar Plexus Chakra

Location: Solar plexus

Purpose: Center of psychic feelings:

Issues associated with your 3rd chakra:

- Personal identity
- Well-balanced energy
- Willpower
- Self-esteem
- Personal achievement
- Balanced ego

If your 3rd chakra is deficient:

- Low energy
- Weak-willed, easily manipulated
- Low self-esteem
- Poor digestion
- Victim mentality
- Poor me
- Passive
- Unreliable
- Easily overwhelmed by others' thoughts and feelings

If your 3rd chakra is excessive:

- Dominating, controlling, overly aggressive
- Need to be right
- Temper tantrums
- Stubborn
- Type A personality
- Arrogant
- Hyperactive

Color: Yellow

Gland: Pancreas

Development age: 18 months to 4 years

Balanced characteristics:

- Responsible, reliable
- Balanced, effective willpower
- Good self-esteem
- Able to feel your feelings
- Able to discern the difference between what you feel and what other people are feeling
- Confident
- Warm
- Relaxed

Physical malfunctions:

- Eating disorders
- Digestive disorders
- Liver, gallbladder, spleen or pancreas problems
- Hypoglycemia or diabetes
- Chronic fatigue
- Muscle spasms

Affirmations:

- I honor who I am and who I have a right to be
- It is safe for me to feel my feelings
- I can do whatever I will to do
- I take pride in my work
- I keep my word
- I respect myself
- I know who I am
- I can say no when I need to

To heal wounds of your 3rd chakra:

- Protect your solar plexus by imagining a screen in front of it
- Visualize energy coming from the crown of your head and pushing out from your 3rd chakra like water pouring out of a fire hydrant

- Express your anger in appropriate ways, *e.g.,* punch a pillow or roll up your car windows and yell
- Ask yourself how you are really feeling
- Take risks
- Deep relaxation, stress management
- Martial arts
- Learn to say no
- Develop your willpower
- Eat yellow fruits and vegetables
- Balance your blood sugar

Sound: Ram, E note

Yoga postures that benefit your 3rd chakra:
- Spinal twists, bow, wheel, bridge, seated boat, lying facing boat, reverse plank, breath of joy, warrior poses, sun salutes

4th Chakra, Anahata, Heart Chakra

Location: Heart center

Purpose: To give and receive love

Issues:

- Love

- Balance
- Self-nurturing
- Relationships
- Devotion
- Reaching out and taking in
- Balance between the physical and spiritual
- Body-mind integration

If the 4th chakra is deficient:

- Withdrawn, cold, antisocial
- Judgmental
- Intolerant of self or others
- Depression
- Loneliness
- Fear of intimacy
- Lack of empathy
- Narcissism

If the 4th chakra is excessive:
- Codependent
- Demanding
- Clinging
- Jealousy
- Overly sacrificing
- Giving too much

Color: Green

Gland: Thymus

Developmental age: 4 to 7 years

Balanced characteristics:

- Compassionate
- Loving
- Empathetic
- Self-loving
- Altruistic
- Peaceful
- Strong immune system
- Happy

Physical malfunctions:

- Heart problems
- Lung problems
- Immune deficiency
- Breathing difficulties
- Circulatory problems
- Tension between shoulder blades

Affirmations:

- I love myself unconditionally
- I am able to give and receive love
- I balance giving and receiving in my life
- I deserve to be loved
- There is an infinite supply of love in my life
- I am the place that love flows through
- I am loving to myself and others
- I love what I do
- I am surrounded by love and support

To heal wounds of your 4th chakra:

- Carry your own baby picture
- Write yourself a love letter
- Eat green fruits and vegetables
- Create a spiritual family of friends who really love you
- Say I am sorry to someone you need to
- Adopt an animal from the pet rescue
- Write a gratitude list
- Work with your arms
- Hug and be hugged
- Forgive yourself and others
- Journal
- Breathing exercises
- Do what you love to do

Sound: Yam, F note

Yoga postures that benefit your 4th chakra:
- Back bends, fish, camel, bridge, wheel, cobra, child, upward facing dog, sage twist, triangle, balancing half moon

5th Chakra, Vissudha, Throat Chakra

Location: Throat center

Purpose: Center for psychic communication

Issues:

- Communication
- Creativity
- Listening
- Finding one's own voice
- Resonation

If the 5th chakra is deficient:

- Fear of speaking your mind
- Small voice
- Tone-deaf
- Shy, introverted
- Difficulty putting your feelings into words

If the 5th chakra is excessive:

- Talk too much
- Unable to listen or understand
- Gossiping
- Dominating voice
- You interrupt others

Color: Blue

Glands: Thyroid, parathyroid

Developmental age: 7 to 12 years

Balanced characteristics:

- Good listener
- Resonant voice
- Good sense of timing and rhythm
- Clear communication
- Creative

Physical malfunctions:

- Thyroid problems
- Disorders of neck, throat, jaws and ears
- Toxicity in the body
- Voice problem

Affirmations:

- I speak my truth with love and grace
- I express myself clearly
- I listen with my whole heart
- I allow my thoughts to flow
- I speak from my heart

To heal wounds of your 5th chakra:

- Play a musical instrument
- Write letters that you later burn and release to the universe
- Practice silence
- Listen to music
- Sing, chant, tone
- Tell stories
- Write in a journal
- Laugh
- Express who you really are
- Eat blue fruits

Sound: Ham, G note

Yoga poses that heal your 5th chakra:
- Shoulderstand, fish, neck stretches, neck rolls, rabbit, plow, knee to ear pose

6th Chakra, Ajna, Third Eye Chakra

Location: Between your eyebrows

Purpose: Psychic vision

Issues:

- Vision
- Intuition
- Imagination
- Visualization
- Insight
- Dreams
- Visions

If your 6th chakra is deficient:

- Insensitivity
- Poor vision
- Poor memory
- Difficulty seeing the future or alternatives
- Lack of imagination
- Difficulty visualizing
- Can't remember dreams
- Denial -- can't see what's really going on

If your 6th chakra is excessive:

- Hallucinations
- Obsessions
- Delusions
- Difficulty concentrating
- Nightmares

Color: Indigo, a blend of red and blue

Gland: Pituitary

Developmental age: Adolescence

Balanced characteristics:

- Intuitive
- Perceptive
- Good memory
- Imaginative
- Able to access and remember dreams
- Able to visualize
- Able to think symbolically

Physical malfunctions:

- Eye problems
- Headaches

Affirmations:

- It is safe for me to see the truth
- My life evolves with clarity
- I honor my psychic vision
- I can manifest my vision
- I am open to the wisdom within
- I imagine wonderful things for my life
- I like what I see

To heal wounds of your 6th chakra:

- Get enough natural sunlight
- Purchase a light-therapy box
- Meditate
- Create visual art -- paint, draw
- Meditate
- Visit art galleries
- Look at beautiful scenery
- Climb to the top of a mountain and enjoy the view
- Always look your best
- Get a makeover
- Surround yourself with beauty
- Use full-spectrum lightbulbs
- Garden

Sound: Om, A note

Yoga postures that benefit 6th chakra:

- Meditation, lotus, yoga mudra, cow's head, dancer, spinal twists, plough, bridge, shoulderstand, eagle

7th chakra, Sahasrara, Crown Chakra

Location: Crown of your head

Purpose: Psychic knowing

Issues:

- Spirituality
- Connection to God
- Transcendence
- Belief systems
- Union
- Wisdom and mastery

If your 7th chakra is deficient:

- Depression
- Spiritual cynicism
- Learning difficulties

- Rigid belief systems
- Apathy

If your 7th chakra is excessive:

- Overly intellectual
- Spiritual addiction
- Confusion
- Disassociation from the body

Color: Violet fading to white

Gland: Pineal

Developmental age: Early adulthood

Balanced characteristics:

- Spiritual outlook on life
- Able to learn easily
- Intelligent, thoughtful, aware
- Open-minded
- Humble before the beauty and wonder of the universe

Physical malfunctions:

- Head injury

- Mental illness
- Coma
- Migraines
- Brain tumors
- Amnesia

Affirmations:

- I honor the divinity within me
- I am connected to God and all that is
- I am guided by my higher power
- I am guided by a higher wisdom
- I honor my knowing
- I follow my inner guidance
- Information I need comes to me whenever I need it
- I am a soul with a physical body
- I am passionate about my life
- I do the best I can
- I am open to new learning
- I accept all parts of myself
- I accept everything that happens in my life as a blessing from God
- I know and experience that I am blessed by God

To heal wounds of your 7th chakra:
- Read spiritual literature
- Attend church, synagogue, or meditate

regularly
- Wear white clothing
- Connect your body, mind and spirit
- Pray
- Attend programs of learning and study
- Listen to the silence
- Use "cancel that" for any negativity
- Practice watching your thoughts
- Talk to God
- Rest one day a week

When you struggle with pain in a particular area of your body, you can begin to heal yourself by nurturing your respective chakra.

Chapter 3. How to Trace Your Acupuncture Meridians for Pain Relief

"The universe doesn't hear what you are saying, it only feels the vibration of what you are offering."
- Abraham-Hicks

If you know how to heal yourself, you feel empowered rather than hopeless when you experience the inevitable pinches and throbs of life.

You can eliminate these discomforts by learning to trace your acupuncture meridians.

You do not have to be a Reiki master, acupuncturist, acupressure expert or any kind of energy healer to be able to do this effectively.

You can get rid of your own aches anytime, anywhere – no drugs, no natural healing remedies, no expensive doctor visits – just you clearing your own energy.

Your Acupuncture Meridians

How does this work?

Whenever you experience pain anywhere in your body, the chi flow in your energy system has been disrupted.

You could have a block on a specific acupuncture meridian. Or you may be experiencing congestion, over energy or under energy in any number of meridians.

Because these energy vessels feed energy into your organs and muscles, if the energy flow in your acupuncture meridians becomes disrupted, your organs and muscles can't function optimally.

By learning to trace your meridians on a daily basis, you can balance the energy in your whole body and relieve much of your pain without drugs.

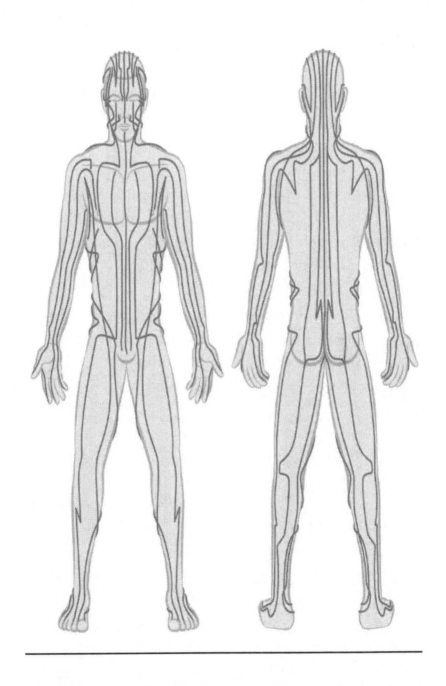

FULL BODY MERIDIANS

Here's how to perform this simple technique:

1. Study the charts above.

2. Pick an acupuncture meridian. Start with the Conception Vessel because it brings energy to your brain and your eyes. This is your primary yin meridian in the body. The Conception Vessel originates in the center of your pubic bone and comes up to the middle of the bottom of your lower lip.

3. Then trace the Governing Vessel, the primary yang meridian of your body. Touch your tailbone and trace up the back of your body above the crown of your head to the top of your upper lip

4. Now turn to your other meridians, which are bilateral meaning they occur on both sides of your body.

5. Take your right hand and touch the beginning of the meridian on the left side of your body

6. Then repeat the process with your left hand touching the beginning of the meridian on your right side.

7. Trace each meridian in the direction of its natural flow. Yin meridians need to be traced upward. The Yin meridians of the arm are Lung, Heart, and Pericardium Meridians. The Yin Meridians of the

leg are Spleen, Kidney, and Liver.

8. Yang Meridians need to be traced downward. The Yang Meridians of the arm are Large Intestine, Small Intestine, and Triple Warmer Meridians. The Yang Meridians of the leg are Stomach, Bladder, and Gall Bladder Meridians.

9. Once you have traced all the other meridians, trace your Conception Vessel and Governing Meridians again to balance the yin and yang energies in your body. Relax and breathe deeply.

If you feel heaviness, congestion, throbbing or other signs of discomfort, you may trace any particular meridian more frequently until you experience relief.

Traditionally you touch the beginning of the meridian, but your hands may pass gently away from your physical body since your energy body generally extends one to three inches outside your skin.

Notice how you feel lighter and more balanced as you progress.

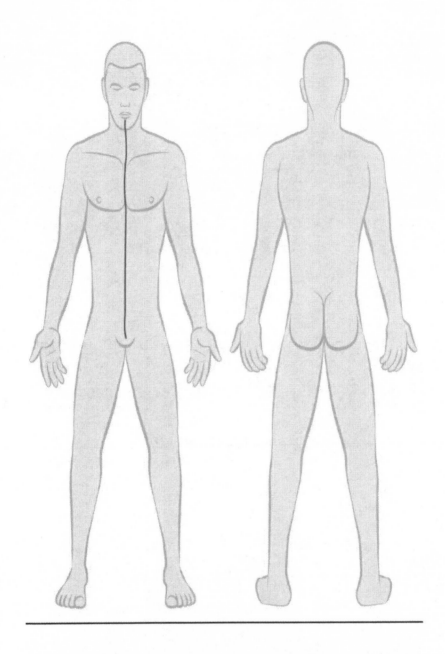

CONCEPTION VESSEL

How To Trace Your Conception Vessel

Directions:
- Touch the center of your pubic bone
- Using the open palm of your hand, trace up the center of your body under the chin just below your lower lip
- Touch the center of your lower lip
- Repeat three times
- Breathe and relax!

Benefits:
- Brings energy to your brain and your eyes
- Balances your primary yin meridian
- Increases chi to your supraspinatus muscles
- Increases your energy

Emotional benefits of a balanced Conception Vessel:
- Self respect
- Success
- Wisdom

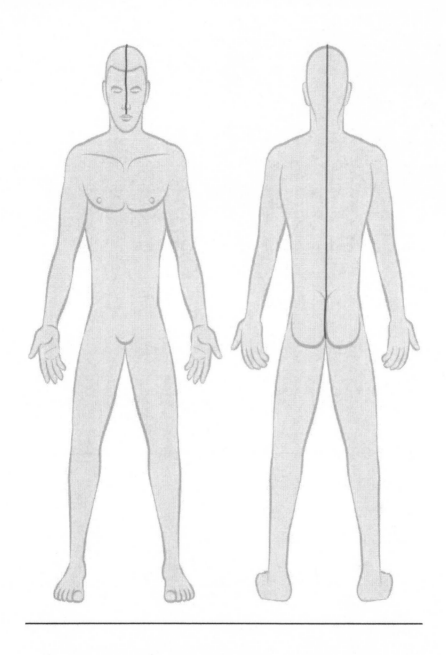

GOVERNING VESSEL

How To Trace Your Governing Vessel

Directions:

- Touch the center of your tail bone
- Using the open palm of your hand, trace up the center of your back, over the top of your head and down your face to the center of your upper lip
- Touch the center of your upper lip
- Repeat three times
- Breathe and relax!

Benefits:
- Helps you feel grounded and supported
- Brings energy to your back
- Increases chi to your teres major muscles
- Balances your primary yang meridian

Emotional benefits of a balanced Governing Vessel:
- You feel supported
- Honesty
- Truthfulness
- Alignment
- Trust
- Living by your values

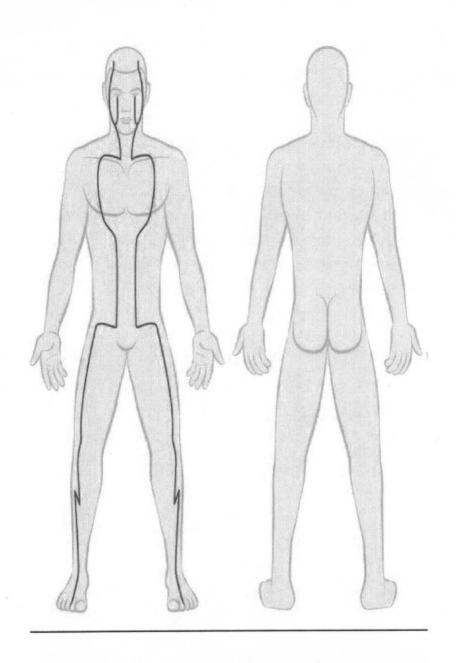

STOMACH MERIDIAN

How To Trace Your Stomach Meridian

Directions:

- From below your eyes, take the open palm of your hand and trace around the cheeks to your forehead and over each eye
- Trace down your jaw
- Continue down your neck and across your collar bone
- Continue down your chest and abdomen
- Cross over the front of your hip
- Go down the outside of the front of your legs to the end of your second toe
- Repeat three times
- Breathe and relax!

Benefits:
- Brings energy to your stomach
- Helps to balance your neck muscles
- Increases chi to your pectoralis major clavicular and brachioradialis muscles

Emotional benefits of a balanced Stomach Meridian:
- Contentment
- Satisfaction
- Sympathy
- Empathy
- Harmony

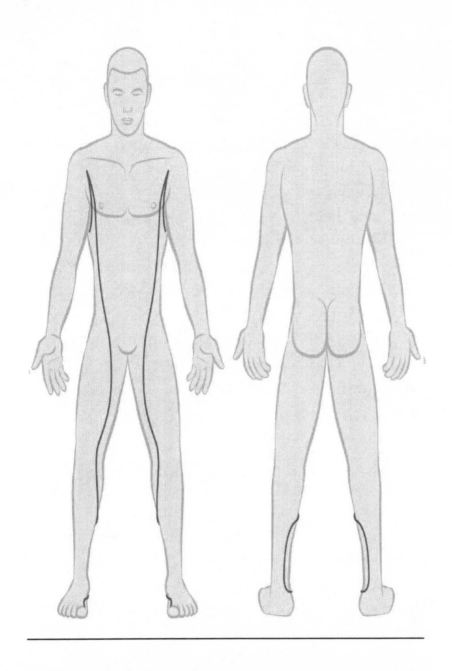

SPLEEN MERIDIAN

How To Trace Your Spleen Meridian

Directions:

- From your big toes, take the open palm of your hand and trace up the inside of your legs
- Continue over the front of your abdomen
- Come up to the side of your chest
- Then trace down your side to below your arm pits
- Repeat three times
- Breathe and relax!

Benefits:
- Brings energy to your spleen
- Increases chi to your latissimus dorsi, trapezius and opponens pollicis longus and triceps muscles

Emotional benefits of a balanced Spleen Meridian:
- Decreased worry
- Reflection
- Assurance
- Faith in the future
- Confidence
- Sympathy

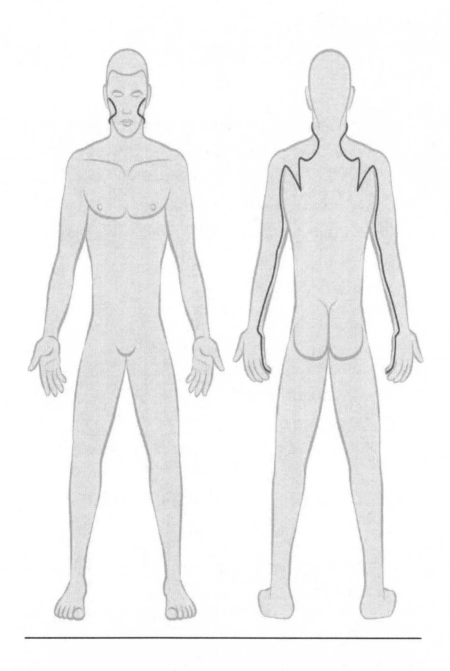

SMALL INTESTINE MERIDIAN

~ 114 ~

How To Trace Your Small Intestine Meridian

Directions:

- From the end of your little finger, trace up the edge of the back of your arm
- Continue to your cheeks
- Trace towards your nose and then back towards the side of your ears
- Repeat three times
- Breathe and relax!

Benefits:
- Brings energy to your small intestines
- Increases chi to your quadriceps and abdominal muscles

Emotional benefits of a balanced Small Intestine Meridian:
- Joy
- Appreciation
- Assimilation of all you learn
- Taking in what you need

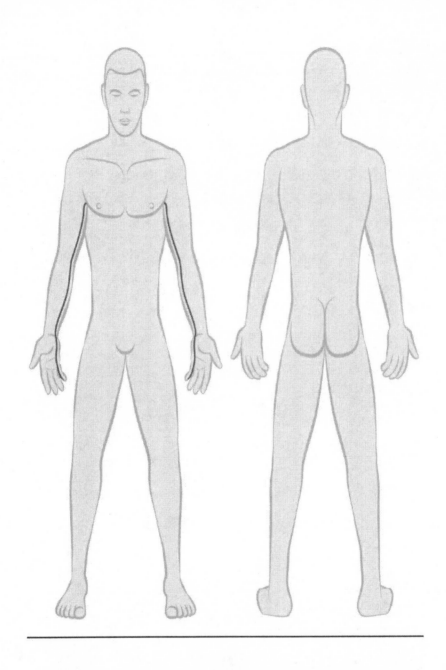

HEART MERIDIAN

How To Trace Your Heart Meridian

Directions:

- From your arm pits, trace down your arm
- Continue to the end of your little finger
- Repeat three times
- Breathe and relax!

Caution:
- Only trace downward
- Never trace your heart meridian backward

Benefits:
- Brings energy to your heart
- Increases chi to your subscapularis muscles

Emotional benefits of a balanced Heart Meridian:
- Love
- Forgiveness
- Compassion
- Knowing who you are
- Self confidence
- Self esteem
- Feeling secure

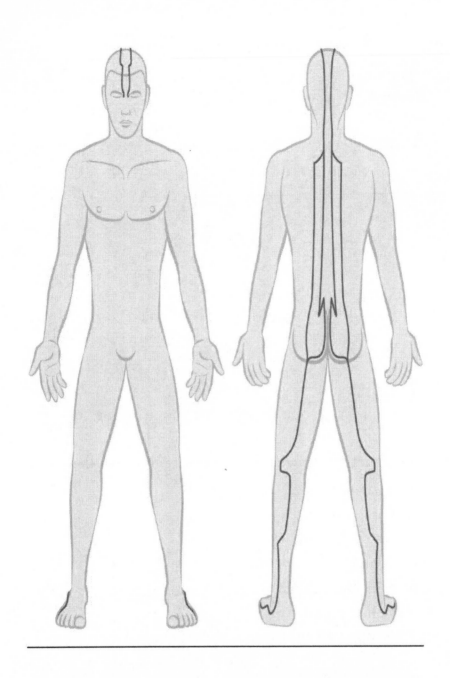

BLADDER MERIDIAN

How To Trace Your Bladder Meridian

Directions:

- From the end of your eyes, trace over your head
- Continue down the back of your body
- Trace along the inside to your buttocks
- Trace back upwards to your shoulders
- Continue down toward the back of your legs
- Touch the end of your little toes
- Repeat three times
- Breathe and relax!

Benefits:
- Brings energy to your bladder
- Increases chi to your tibials, peroneus and sacrospinalis muscles

Emotional benefits of a balanced Small Intestine Meridian:
- Feeling in charge of your own life
- Not needing to be a control freak
- Peace
- Inner direction
- Confidence
- Courage
- Patience

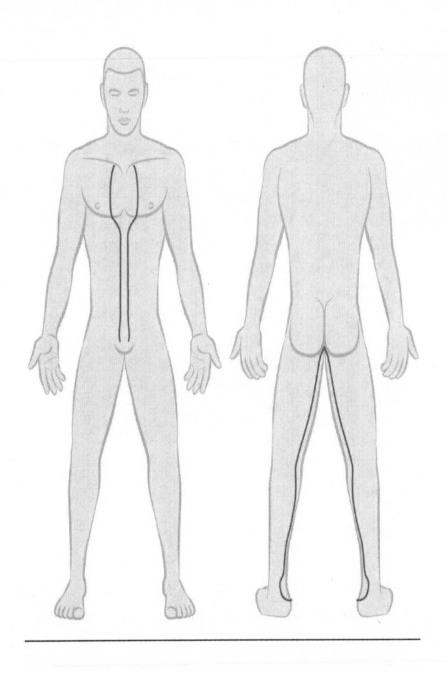

KIDNEY MERIDIAN

How To Trace Your Kidney Meridian

Directions:

- From the ball of your foot, trace up the inside of your leg
- Continue to your abdomen and chest
- Touch the knobs on your collar bones
- Repeat three times
- Breathe and relax!

Benefits:
- Brings energy to your kidneys
- Increases chi to your psoas, iliacus and upper trapezius muscles

Emotional benefits of a balanced Kidney Meridian:
- Balanced sexual energy
- Feeling sexually secure
- Feeling creatively secure
- Giving your whole spirit to life
- Trusting your process

Special note:
- Unfortunately this image is a little confusing, making it appear as if the kidney meridian is split in two. It's actually one meridian.

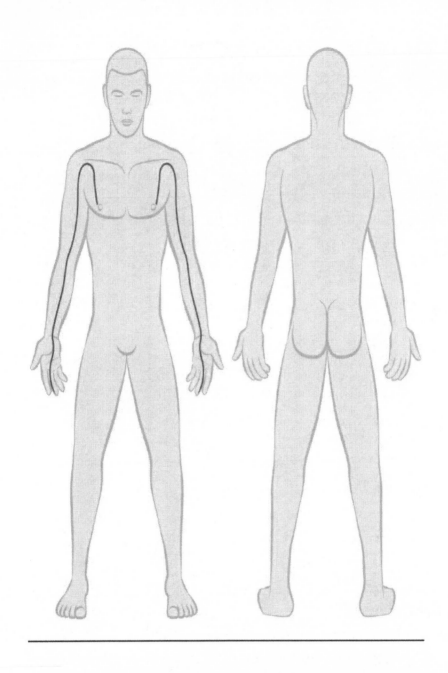

PERICARDIUM MERIDIAN

~ 122 ~

How To Trace Your Pericardium Meridian

Directions:

- From your nipples, trace down the middle of the inside of your arms
- Continue to the end of each middle finger
- Repeat three times
- Breathe and relax!

Benefits:
- Brings energy to your heart
- Increases chi to your gluteus medius, adductors, piriformis and gluteus maximus muscles

Emotional benefits of a balanced Pericardium Meridian:
- Feeling connected
- Bonding
- Forgiveness
- Tranquility
- Responsibility
- Calmness
- Relaxation

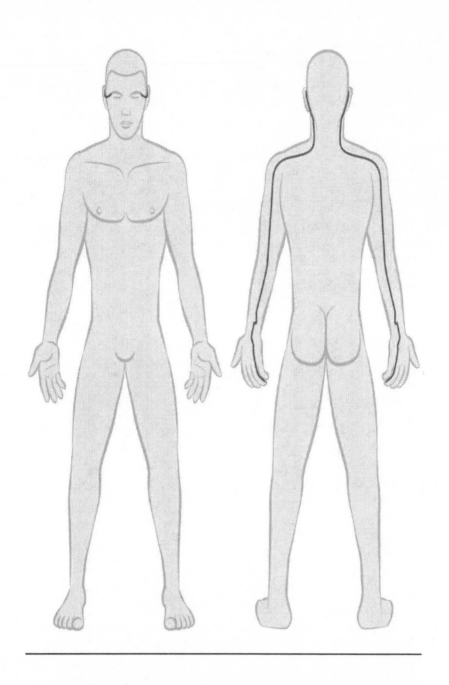

TRIPLE WARMER MERIDIAN

How To Trace Your Triple Warmer Meridian

Directions:

- From the end of your ring fingers, trace up the back of your hand
- Continue up the back of your arm to the side of your neck
- Go around the back of your ears
- Touch just outside your eyebrows
- Repeat three times
- Breathe and relax!

Benefits:
- Brings energy to your thyroid and adrenal glands
- Increases chi to your teres minor, sartorius, gastrocnemius and gracilis muscles

Emotional benefits of a balanced Triple Warmer Meridian:
- Feeling in harmony with the flow of life
- Elation
- Lightness
- Hope
- Balance
- Buoyancy
- Solitude

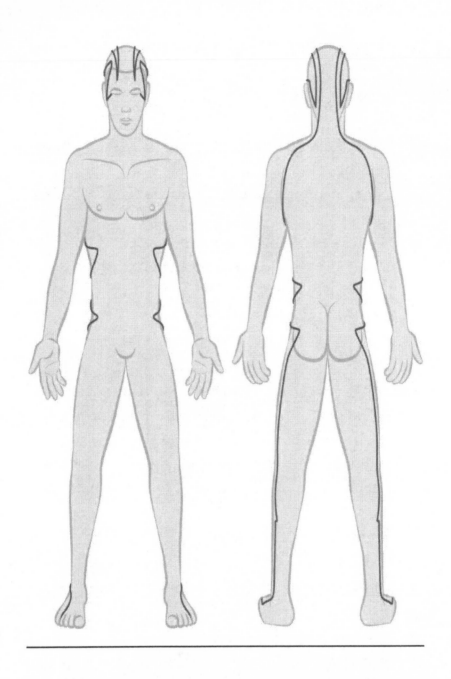

GALL BLADDER MERIDIAN

How To Trace Your Gall Bladder Meridian

Directions:

- From the corner of your eyes, loop around the side of your forehead
- Go behind your ears to your forehead down the back of your head
- Continue down the back of your shoulder under your arms
- Go down the side of your chest and the outside of your leg
- Touch the end of your fourth toe
- Repeat three times
- Breathe and relax!

Benefits:
- Brings energy to your gall bladder
- Increases chi to your anterior deltoid and popliteus muscles

Emotional benefits of a balanced Gall Bladder Meridian:
- Able to make choices that are right for you and in the entire universe
- Love
- Motivation
- Assertive
- Humility
- Pride

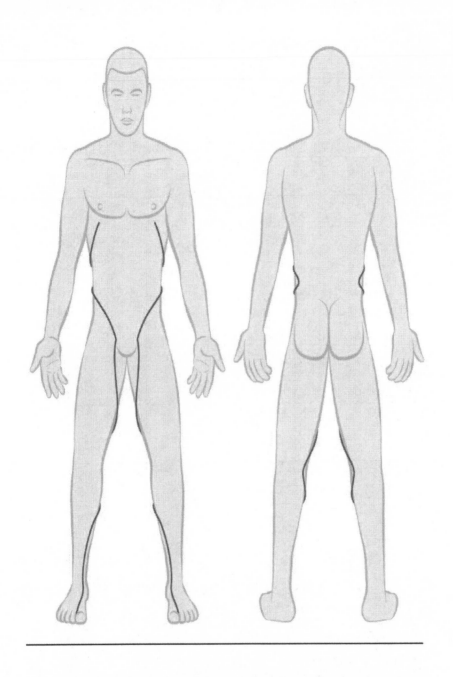

LIVER MERIDIAN

How To Trace Your Liver Meridian

Directions:

- From inside your big toes, trace up the inside of your legs to your hips
- Go wide around your waist
- Then continue inward toward your chest
- Repeat three times
- Breathe and relax!

Benefits:
- Brings energy to your liver
- Increases chi to your pectoralis major sternal and rhomboid muscles

Emotional benefits of a balanced Liver Meridian:
- Creativity
- Happiness
- Transformation

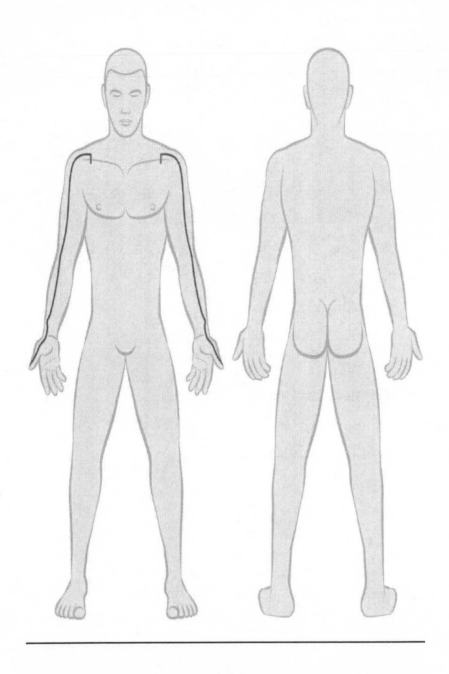

LUNG MERIDIAN

How To Trace Your Lung Meridian

Directions:

- From just above your lungs, trace down the outside of the front of your arms
- Continue to the end of your thumbs
- Repeat three times
- Breathe and relax!

Benefits:
- Brings energy to your lungs
- Increases chi to your anterior serratus, coracobrachialis and diaphragm muscles

Emotional benefits of a balanced Lung Meridian:
- Self worth
- Humility
- Cheerfulness
- Tolerance
- Openness
- Modesty

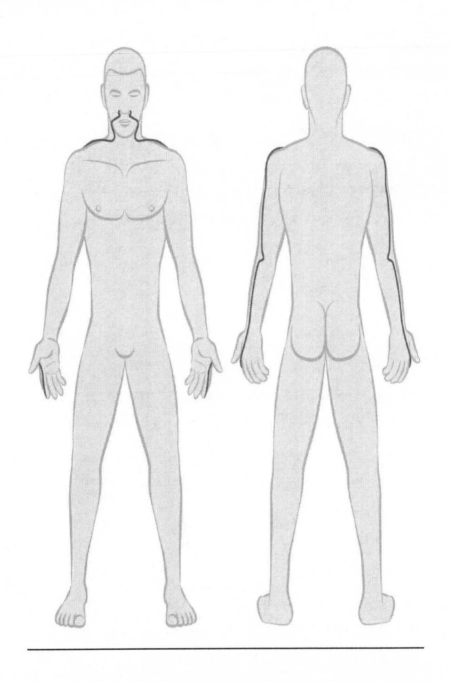

LARGE INTESTINE MERIDIAN

How To Trace Your Large Intestine Meridian

Directions:

- From the end of your index fingers, trace up the outside of the back of your hands
- Continue up your arms
- Continue up your neck to your lower lip
- End at the side of your nose
- Repeat three times
- Breathe and relax!

Benefits:
- Brings energy to your large intestine
- Increases chi to your fascia lata, hamstrings and quadratus lumborum muscles

Emotional benefits of a balanced Large Intestine Meridian:
- Letting go
- Self worth
- Compassion
- Release of the past
- Making space for beneficial change

Chapter 4. Heal Your Neck and Shoulder Pain Naturally

"We are not just highly evolved animals with biological computers embedded inside our skulls; we are also fields of consciousness without limits, transcending time, space, matter and linear causality."
- Stanislav Grof

Wouldn't you like to learn how to get rid of neck and shoulder pain naturally, without having to go to the chiropractor, get a massage or even do any stretching?

That's exactly what we did in my qi gong class recently.
I taught everybody how to release the Triple Warmer Meridian.

I frequently interrupt the exercise portion of the class to teach simple, quick energy-healing techniques. That way my students learn how to heal themselves anytime, anywhere, with no equipment.

Many people give up hope because they don't understand how their body really works. They don't understand their metabolism, energy system, muscles or what will actually work to make them better.

One of my qi gong students told me that when she came to class, her neck and shoulder pain were at a level of 5 out of 10 with zero being no pain.

After doing the Triple Warmer Meridian release, she had NO pain!

Triple Warmer Release

Step One. Put your hands on either side of the outer edge of your eyebrows. Trace a simple arcing line down to the outside of your ears. Repeat. Keep flushing with both hands, brushing from the outside of the eyebrows to the ears.

Step Two. Trace from the outside of the eyebrows to in front of the ears and then trace over the ears. Repeat. Keep flushing with both hands, brushing from the eyebrows to the ears and over the ears.

Step Three. Now trace from the outside of the eyebrows to in front of the ears to over the ears and then down to the back of your shoulders. Repeat.

What you will feel: As you pass your hands, you will probably feel a tingling sensation and increased relaxation.

How this works: This exercise flushes the Triple Warmer Meridian. When you are stressed, this meridian steals chi from other meridians in the body. You may notice that your shoulders are tightening up and riding up closer to your ears.

The triple heater is also called the San Jiao Meridian. On an emotional level, it has to do with being in harmony. Are you in harmony with yourself? Are you in harmony with the world around you?

You can use these affirmations:

I am in harmony with the flow of life. I go with the flow.

I flow with grace and ease through all changes in my life.

I am in harmony with my true self. My body naturally reflects my true self. My body naturally reflects my inner harmony.

I am in harmony inside and out, outside and in on all levels now in an easy and healthy way.

Most of the time to be in harmony, you need to slow down and get in touch with how you really feel at the soul level.

Chapter 5. Eight Minutes to Inner Peace

"Our breathing reflects every emotional or physical effort and every disturbance."
- Moshe Feldenkrais

You can release the distressing energy trapped inside you by practicing this powerful yoga breathing sequence. I have taught this routine to countless clients suffering from anxiety, depression, high blood pressure, asthma, chronic obstructive pulmonary disease, kidney failure, insomnia and many other ailments.

What if all you had to do was breathe away your pain? Try it now!

Start by sitting or lying down in a comfortable position.

- ONE MINUTE: Focus on lengthening your inhale.

- ONE MINUTE: Focus on lengthening your exhale.

- ONE MINUTE: Focus on making your inhale and exhale equally long and deep.

Sit up for the remaining breathing exercises.

- ONE MINUTE: Bellows Breath. Inhale into your belly and exhale forcibly by contracting your solar plexus.

- ONE MINUTE: Breath of Fire. While inhaling and exhaling rapidly, pump your diaphragm. Your inhale will happen naturally.

- ONE MINUTE: Alternate Nostril Breathing. Inhale through your right nostril. With the thumb of your right hand, close the right nostril. Exhale through your left nostril. With the ring finger of your right hand, close the left nostril. Exhale through your right nostril. Use your thumb to close your right nostril. Exhale through the left nostril. Use your ring finger to close the left. Repeat.

- ONE MINUTE: Bumblebee Breath. Place your pointer finger and middle finger on your forehead. Place your thumbs on your earflaps and close your ears. Place your ring finger lightly on your closed eyelids, letting your little finger rest on your cheekbones. Make a humming sound like a bee.

- ONE MINUTE: Ocean Breath. Open your mouth, relax your jaw. Inhale and make the sound of the ocean in the back of your throat. Exhale and make the sound of the ocean. Close your lips and continue making the sound of the ocean.

When you are finished, notice how your mind has moved into a peaceful, meditative state. Give yourself permission to sit quietly or lie down and enjoy feeling fabulous!

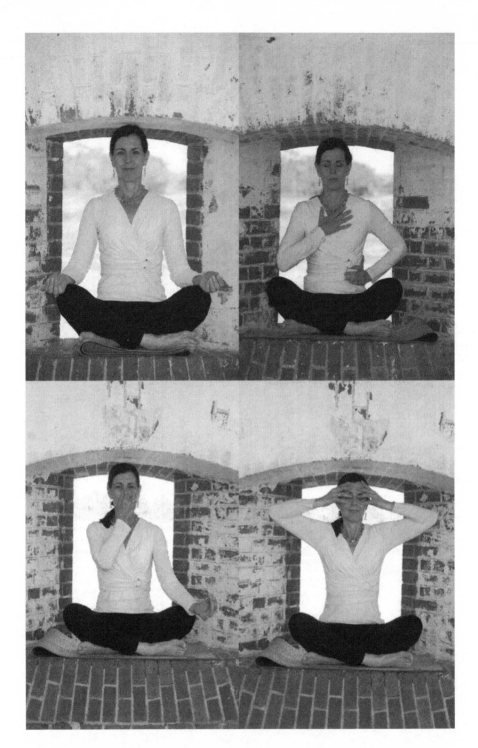

Chapter 6. Repair the Holes in Your Energy Field

"I know this transformation is painful, but you're not falling apart; you're just falling into something different, with a new capacity to be beautiful."
- William C. Hannan

One of the ways to make the biggest difference in your overall health and well-being is to repair the holes in your energy field.

What is your energy field? Your human energy field, also known as your auric field, is the field of energy wrapping around your physical body. It's a law of physics that any vertical electrical current has a magnetic field perpendicular to it.

Your entire body is electrical. Medical doctors can measure your EKG from your heart and your EEG from your brain.

Those of us who practice energy exercise such as yoga, tai chi and qi gong strengthen and expand our auric field. But your auric field may experience tears. Some of the tears I have repaired over the years include:

- A young man who had been raped by three men

- A woman who had suffered a diving accident

- Numerous clients who had experienced chronic back pain not alleviated by chiropractic treatments, massage or other natural healing techniques

- A fellow healer who had been suffering from obsessive compulsive disorder (OCD) and searching for two years for another healer to help her

So why is repairing the tears in your energy field so crucial? Let me tell you a story.

Recently a young woman came to me after being raped. She was referred to me by one of my regular clients.

"I heard her story and immediately gave her your phone number," my client said. "She had so many things wrong that I knew you were the only person who could really help her."

When she came into my office, I explained that the first thing I was going to do was to remove the shock and trauma from her body.

It was not her fault she had been raped. She had gone to a party, thought she was drinking a Sprite and ended up awaking the next morning with bruises all over her body.

The doctors at the hospital determined she had been given a date rape drug that included a horse tranquilizer. She had no memory of who had raped her. It appeared she must have put up a fight as the front door to her apartment had been damaged.

When she came to me, she reported experiencing panic, night terrors and severe depression not alleviated by heavy psychiatric medication.

"My doctor told me I have post-traumatic stress disorder (PTSD) as bad as a person who has shell shock from a mortar injury," she told me.

First, I removed the negative spiritual energy. That means I removed the low vibrational frequencies that had attached to her during the rape.

Then I checked her energy grid. I found a huge hole in the back of her auric field and used Reiki healing energy to repair it.

The tear was probably about six inches by six inches around her thoracic spine. It was no surprise she had been experiencing unrelenting pain there.
Then I removed the energetic residue of the date rape drug.

Finally, I took her nervous system out of shock. She had been holding the feeling of panic in her left hip and left knee.

Previously she had gone four nights without sleeping.

By taking her out of shock, I restored balance between her sympathetic and parasympathetic nervous systems.

"You may be quite tired after this healing," I explained.

"By restoring balance to your nervous system, you will finally be able to relax."

Years ago, a young man had been referred to me by his school guidance counselor. He had been over-exercising to the point of collapse and had to be taken away by ambulance not just once but several times.

No one really knew what was going on with him.

I was only the second person he talked to about the fact he had been raped.

One afternoon his mother had been late to pick him up from theater practice, and three men jumped him. He was so embarrassed he held it in for two years.

"You can't fix this yourself," I explained.

I repaired the huge hole in the back of his auric field.

At our next visit, he told me, "I know you know you helped me, but you have no idea how much you helped me."

I was glad to hear he was feeling so much better but shocked and upset when his mother called the very next day and canceled our future sessions.

"She wants to save money," he explained in an e-mail. He did not want to admit to his mother what had happened because he did not want her to feel guilty.

Had he been under the age of 18, I would have been legally required to report the incident to the police. I honored his confidentiality but struggled to communicate to his mother that he still desperately needed help.

She ignored my pleas. For me, this was an extreme lesson in being able to honor a person's spiritual path, knowing that God takes care of all of us and leads us exactly to what we need. I still pray for this young man as well as his family.

Another woman I helped had suffered a diving accident as a teenager.

Before she became my client, she had been in a one-year study for back pain at the National Institutes of Health, taken Vioxx and even become a Pilates instructor to try to alleviate her suffering.

It wasn't until I repaired the tears in her auric field that her pain went away and she was finally able to take herself off Vioxx.

The largest hole I have ever repaired was in the energy field of the fellow healer who had been experiencing OCD. She walked around with baggies full of tissue paper and wiped her hands incessantly. She even hid plastic baggies full of the tissues around my garden.

Even though she had visited countless other healers, it wasn't until I patched the hole in her auric field that she began to experience relief.

If you have experienced trauma, please be aware that you may have torn holes in your auric field. If this is the case, you may have the following symptoms:

- PTSD
- Migraines
- Pain and suffering not alleviated by medication
- Anxiety and depression

- Sensitivity to energy
- Multiple chemical sensitivity and environmental sensitivity

If you have tears to your energy field, there are several ways to repair it:

- Visit a highly trained energy healer.
- Practice tai chi, qi gong and/or yoga, which restores balance to the energy field around your body.

What works to overcome pain and suffering? Healing happens when you patch the holes in your auric field.

Chapter 7. The Magic of Eights

"Each day you must choose the pain of discipline or the
pain of regret."
- Eric Mangini

You can relieve pain anytime, anywhere, by using the
magic of eights. Figure-eight patterns work because of
the way energy flows in your body.

Energy flows up the Central Acupuncture Meridian.
Then it flows over to the left, circling down and then up
again through the Central Meridian, over to the right,
down around and up again through the same meridian.

This is a lazy-eight pattern – an eight lying on its side.

Years ago, one of my clients was a landscaper.

She asked me to help her move some rocks.

When I saw the "rocks," I realized she was wanting me
to help her move *boulders*!

We went to a creek and were trying to pick up these
boulders when, by accident, I smashed my middle finger.
I could tell immediately it was broken.

The first thing I did, while standing in the creek bed,

was to use my other hand to make figure-eight patterns over the broken finger. I could feel the energy release every time I made the figure eight over the swelling finger.

I continued to make figure eights as we walked back to my client's house, where I put my hand in a bowl of ice water and began making phone calls to the hospital.

This is a very important technique to learn if you happen to be alone or out of the reach of traditional therapies when you hurt yourself. Even if no other tools are available, you can use figure eights to relieve your pain.

In a qi gong class recently, I taught a series of exercises based on figure eights. By moving your body in figure-eight patterns, you can balance the gallbladder, stomach, small intestine and lung meridians. We also performed natural vision improvement exercises using figure-eight patterns.

Then I taught my class how to use figure eights with hands-on healing. We lined up in a straight line and drew figure eights on each other's backs. I was at the end of the line directing the movement. Everyone could feel their backs relax.

Then we drew figure eights around each other's adrenal glands – the glands on top of your kidneys that secrete stress hormones. As each person was drawing the figure eights, I had them visualize the color gold.

Gold is the most healing color. There are many healing benefits to all colors of the rainbow, as each acupuncture meridian, organ and chakra responds to particular frequencies. But gold is the highest frequency of the aura and arguably the most therapeutic color.

If you use figure eights as a healing technique, you should muscle-test or ask for guidance about which direction to draw your eight over an affected area.

You can draw figure eights on the bottoms of your feet, on your hands, on the core of your body, on the top of your head.

Drawing figure eights balances the energy flow in your body. You will feel calmer and more relaxed, and any pain will magically diminish.

Chapter 8. What Is Cardiac Low Back?

"We are our choices."
- J.P. Sartre

Cardiac low back is a common condition in which your low back gives out to force you to slow down and keep you from having a heart attack.

When you experience any symptom, your body is signaling to you that something is out of balance.

One of my long-term clients used to run one of the most successful MRI testing facilities in the Atlanta area. She reported to me that low back pain was the No. 1 reason people went to her company's doctors for MRIs, often thinking there must be something structurally wrong with their spine.

As a yoga teacher with 21 years of experience, I can attest that structural imbalances are often the root cause of back pain. I have helped countless clients clear their long-term back pain with an individualized stretching and strengthening program. You can learn the exercises I teach most often for therapeutic purposes by consulting the appendix in the back of this book.

Another major cause of low back pain is simply exhaustion. You are so exhausted that your low back gives out to make you pause, stop and rest to keep the stress off your heart.

You have to ask yourself, is your low back pain trying to tell you something important?

Cardiac low back syndrome can occur even if you exercise regularly and maintain strong core muscles. Why is this the case?

Your heart is the emperor of your body. When you are completely healthy and happy, you enjoy a strong physical heart and exude confidence, courage and passion.

In our society, however, burnout is unfortunately the norm, not the exception. That's why I wrote my book, *Unlimited Energy Now.*

The most common condition I see in all my new clients is chronic, unrelenting fatigue. When your adrenal glands – the tiny glands that sit on top of your kidneys and secrete the stress hormones cortisol and adrenalin – have burned out from years of unresolved stress, your heart reflects this depletion, and you may experience a multitude of symptoms, including low back pain.

Your adrenal glands go through three stages of stress – alarm, adaptation and exhaustion.

You may not even recognize how exhausted you are, but your heart definitely does, and your low back will often reflect how depleted you really feel.

How do you correct cardiac low back? At the end of the day, you will want to commit to life-regenerating practices to rebuild your personal chi.

This may include therapeutic rest, meditation, hot baths, massage, Reiki, qi gong, tai chi, yoga, improved nutrition and reducing your overall stress.

The fastest, cheapest way to overcome adrenal burnout is to take time off and meditate, nap and sleep as much as possible.

What works to overcome pain and suffering? Healing happens when you honor the wisdom of your body and heed its many cries for rest.

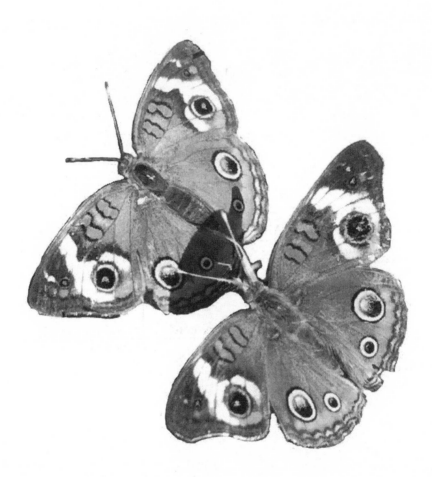

Book IV

Your Emotional Body

Chapter 1. How to Get Out of Hell Without Really Trying

"The only time we suffer is when we believe a thought that argues with what is. When the mind is perfectly clear, what is is what we want."
- Byron Katie

Every once in a while, you make a seriously wrong turn in life and end up in considerable pain.

Because you are in fact divinely loved, even in the depths of your misery, you can be comforted by the fact that torment isn't actually God's will for you. Nowhere in any spiritual text does it read, "Thou shalt suffer."

No, in fact God's will for you is perfect happiness. It's just that sometimes we forget and end up thrashing against our higher nature, against *what is*, fighting the divine wisdom of it all.

Here are two good ways to get out of hell without really trying:

The two percent solution. Often we feel so completely stuck that no relief seems possible. Your head throbs. You're hanging onto the toilet bowl, ready to heave. You hate your job, can't stand your life, and it seems there's no reason to put up with any of it. So ask yourself a simple question: "If I could make my life two percent easier right now, what would I do differently?" You make an infinitesimal shift, so small, so easy, so completely effortless it's almost like you're not really even trying. Make a choice that requires virtually no effort. You take a right turn instead of a left. You stop crossing your legs and sit up straight for a second. You exercise one minute, not one hour. You count to one and then start swearing. You eat one fewer bites of food. You take one deep breath. You do one stretch. Just by taking one teeny-weeny step, you come to realize that you can make yourself feel that much better. And when you recognize that you can make yourself feel even a bit more comfortable, you open up the space for miracles to occur. You create a crack of hope. You get a glimpse of another possibility.

Take your power back. While you are sitting there aching in agony, in your mind, between your ears, ask yourself another simple question: "Where oh where did I give my power away?" You may not even recognize that you did this. Did you drink the Kool-Aid and believe your diagnosis, giving your power away to your doctor? Maybe you gave your power away to your mother, father, husband, wife, boyfriend, girlfriend, brother, sister, aunt, uncle, son, daughter, boss, employee -- somebody who told you something bad about yourself and you believed them. It was so long ago and so subtle that you never even recognized at the time what happened. Where, pray tell, did you drop your personal capacity to be in charge of your own life? Now take your power back. When you do so, you can take your life back. You get to decide who you are, what you should be when you grow up, your very experience of every moment. You are actually in charge. You get to name it, own it, buy it or not buy it. In your mind's eye, when you see the person or situation where you gave your power away, call on the strength of your soul and pull your power back all the way into yourself. Instead of an inch, this second approach may provide a humongous leap forward.

Healing happens when you recognize that you can choose a different way of being.

Chapter 2. What Happens When You Get Stuck in the Pain

"The moment you change your perception is the moment you rewrite the chemistry of your body."
- Bruce Lipton

Because we are all human, sometimes we get stuck in our pain.

In mid-July 2017, my dog Belle died. Just the week before she passed away, I remember thinking, "I don't think I've ever been so happy in my entire life."

Then one Monday afternoon we were out in my garden beside the zinnias and Belle walked off a four-foot-high wall, falling onto the concrete below without so much as a whimper.

She was just an arm's length away, but I was unable to save her.

I screamed and ran to her, hugging her, trying to reassure her.

That night a friend drove us to the vet's office.

The vet shined a light into Belle's eyes, and she didn't react. The quick diagnosis: She was blind.

My brother, an ophthalmologist, had examined Belle's eyes just a few weeks before and correctly pinpointed the problem.

"She has a brain tumor," my brother told me. "There's nothing you can do. You need to put her down."

It was true Belle had been falling down the stairs of late, all the way down the wooden steps from the top floor to the second floor, to the point I had been making a habit of carrying her around in my arms to keep her from hurting herself. In fact, I had been carrying Belle around so much that my arms habitually ached.

I prayed for guidance. That night I held Belle close, petting her, comforting her, holding her sweet soft body as if I was trying to imprint her very being into every cell of my own.

The next morning Belle remained silent as we drove to the vet for the last time.

I held her in my arms as she received the final injection. It was I who was sobbing, not Belle.

The vet techs came and wrapped little Belle's suddenly lifeless body in a black blanket. They handed me her leash and harness as I sat there completely bereft.

The rest of the day I could hardly eat. My head throbbed.

I scheduled a visit for craniosacral therapy and then lay on the floor of the yoga room in my house afterwards weeping, inert.

There was nothing anyone could say or do to make me feel better.

A few days later, I was driving my Prius down the road near my house when I suddenly veered to the right and got my wheels stuck in a ditch.

A single-car accident.

I can't remember the last time I had a car wreck, and this one cost me more than $700.

"This week was like winning the lottery in reverse," I told my family.

About a week later, I was helping my brother carry a heavy cooler when I accidentally kicked myself. My left big toe started bleeding uncontrollably as the toenail cracked off.

"Done!" I pronounced silently to myself.

All week people had been helpfully pointing out to me that bad luck runs in threes. Holding onto my left big toe, I felt a small sense of relief knowing that the string of unfortunate events had now come to this ignominious end.

All week, my sisters-in-law had been recommending that I eat more food. I would go off into my bedroom to cry for hours. All I could do was live through the process, not really knowing how I could ever let go of all of the grief.

At times like this, it's normal and natural to want relief, usually as soon as humanly possible, even if there doesn't seem to be any way out.

I knew I wasn't going to feel right until I got another dog. And soon enough, God blessed me with a new cocker spaniel named Dixie, a fluffy black and white being who brightens every day of my life.

I am always saying that the quickest way through the mud is *through* the mud -- not over the mud, around the mud, pretending the mud doesn't exist, ignoring the mud or wishing it wasn't in fact right there smack-dab in front of you.

All we can do sometimes is practice compassion for our own humanity, holding ourselves gently in mind as the most precious soul that we are, giving ourselves a pass and not really expecting anything.

As sure as the rain comes, so eventually does the sunshine, if only we sit with ourselves long enough to allow the dark clouds to pass.

Chapter 3. Why Poor Me Doesn't Get Well

"Only I can change my life. No one can do it for me."
- Carol Burnett

One of the most important things you can ever do to get out of pain is to stop playing Poor Me.

Who exactly is Poor Me?

Poor Me is the shadow side of your personality who is always talking about being too busy, too tired, who has lots of problems while everybody else has this easy time of everything. Poor Me struggles along while everybody else gets all the luck, all the money, all the breaks.

Another name for Poor Me could be Debbie Downer, Kevin Killjoy or Pissy Peter.

These evil twin aspects of you could crash your party on the same day you win the lottery, get married, or find out you just got promoted and received a raise.

Just one glance or a small, backhanded comment could be all that it takes.

We all have these little sub personalities who take over our mind and body at times.

Let me give you a good example.

The other day I was talking on Skype with a client who lives near San Francisco. While I was busy focusing on my client for a medical intuitive reading, my little puppy Dixie kept bringing me her tennis balls, scratching my desk and whining. "Isn't it STILL all about me?" my dog seemed to be asking.

Meanwhile, I kept apologizing to my client.

Nobody has ever called me tough especially when it comes to my own puppy. "Pushover" is more like it.

"You have to ask yourself, 'Who has the body?'" I explained to my client. "For example, my puppy's Inner Brat currently has taken charge."

My client nodded her head. "I get it!" she exclaimed.

There's your true self, and then there may be multiple sub personalities that keep you from experiencing radiant health: Inner Brat. Overeater. Lazy Bones Jones. Compulsive Worrier.

One of the worst of these personalities for sure is Poor Me. You will know Poor Me has taken over your body when:

- All you talk about is how busy and tired you are.

- You complain a lot.

- You see the glass as half-empty, practically empty or empty.

- You forget your blessings.

- You destroy any positive energy around you.

- You think everybody else has a leg up on life.

- You have an excuse for everything.

- You find something wrong in any situation.

- You see plenty of reasons why you can't possibly get any better.

- You think other people got a break somehow and you didn't.

- You want other people to accommodate how sick, tired, poor, uncomfortable or disadvantaged you are. Everybody else obviously has it so good they need to alter their lives to make up for what you don't have.

So here's an uncomfortable truth: Poor Me takes you out of your power.

To get out of pain, you have to be *in* your power.

You have to take responsibility for everything that has ever happened to you, including the entire cast of characters in your personal melodrama and how and why you ended up exactly where you are today.

When you are in your power, you find a way.

When you are in your power, you find solutions, not excuses.

When you are in your power, you see yourself as unbreakable, limitless, strong and connected to the benevolent reservoir of all good things otherwise commonly known as God.

You recognize that the universe is in fact a friendly place and that all events conspire for your highest good. You acknowledge that it's all good because it is in fact all God.

You open yourself to possibilities because you see that your entire life is already a miracle. The fact that you made it this far has occurred solely through divine grace, and you consider yourself lucky enough to still be breathing

You say "thank you" for the blessings even when you don't really understand how what's happening could possibly be any good for you.

But you're open to the grace, open to God, open to the friendliness, the benevolence, the miracles, the blessings. It's easy to overlook your blessings when you just got raped, when you just left the rehab center, when you're down to your last $100, when you just got fired. These are the times when you need to do yourself the biggest favor and pay strict attention when Poor Me tries to show up.

It's called tough love, but the mental discipline required to see yourself as whole and always connected to workable solutions is better than sinking into hopelessness.

You have to acknowledge that Poor Me is not here to do you any favors.

What works to overcome pain and suffering? Tell Poor Me to take a hike, and embrace your limitless soul power.

Chapter 4. How Emotions Affect Your Muscles

"Unexpressed emotions will never die. They are buried alive and will come forth later in uglier ways."
- Sigmund Freud

When you feel a pain in the neck, is it really a problem with your cervical vertebrae or your anterior or posterior neck flexors, or have you simply gotten stuck in your emotions?

In other words, do you really have a crick in your neck or a strain in your life? Or both?

Your body speaks the language of emotions. We have to understand that our physical bodies simply respond to what's happening to our energy system, emotions, thoughts and spiritual experience.

You can think of your body like one big hologram with each aspect reflecting what's happening inside and out, above and below, from the cell level to the organ level and beyond.

By the time you experience discomfort in your physical body, you've been grappling with the emotion behind it for some time – even if you haven't been consciously aware.

You may not realize how emotional your body really is until you start to connect the relative ease or discomfort you have been experiencing with the emotions you've been feeling.

Pain in and of itself is an emotion. Can you hear what your body is asking for?

Use the following list to understand your emotional anatomy.

Emotions Affecting Each Major Muscle

Central Meridian

Supraspinatus. Central Acupuncture Meridian. Self-Respect. Overwhelm. Shyness. Success. Shame.

Governing Meridian

Teres Major. Governing Meridian. Embarrassment. Support. Harmony. Trust. Truth.

Stomach Meridian

Pectoralis Major Clavicular. Stomach Meridian. Unreliable. Criticism. Contentment. Disappointment. Deprivation. Hunger. Nausea. Greed. Empty. Sympathy. Empathy. Harmony. Disgust. Doubt. Bitter.

Levator Scapulae. Stomach Meridian. Unreliable. Criticism. Contentment. Disappointment. Deprivation. Hunger. Nausea. Greed. Empty. Sympathy. Empathy. Harmony. Disgust. Doubt. Bitter.

Anterior Neck Flexors. Stomach Meridian. Unreliable. Criticism. Contentment. Disappointment. Deprivation. Hunger. Nausea. Greed. Empty. Sympathy. Empathy. Harmony. Disgust. Doubt. Bitter.

Posterior Neck Extensors. Stomach Meridian. Unreliable. Criticism. Contentment. Disappointment. Deprivation. Hunger. Nausea. Greed. Empty. Sympathy. Empathy. Harmony. Disgust. Doubt. Bitter.

Brachioradialis. Stomach Meridian. Unreliable. Criticism. Contentment. Disappointment. Deprivation. Hunger. Nausea. Greed. Empty. Sympathy. Empathy. Harmony. Disgust. Doubt. Bitter.

Spleen Meridian

Latissimus Dorsi. Spleen Meridian. Rejected. Assurance. Indifference. Disapproval. Faith in the future. Anxiety regarding the future. Consideration. Recollection. Confidence. Alienation. Sympathy. Empathy. Brooding. Cynicism. Envy.

Middle and Lower Trapezius. Spleen Meridian. Rejected. Assurance. Indifference. Disapproval. Faith in the future. Anxiety regarding the future. Consideration. Recollection. Confidence. Alienation. Sympathy. Empathy. Brooding. Cynicism. Envy.

Opponens Pollicis. Spleen Meridian. Rejected. Assurance. Indifference. Disapproval. Faith in the future. Anxiety regarding the future. Consideration. Recollection. Confidence. Alienation. Sympathy. Empathy. Brooding. Cynicism. Envy.

Triceps. Spleen Meridian. Rejected. Assurance. Indifference. Disapproval. Faith in the future. Anxiety regarding the future. Consideration. Recollection. Confidence. Alienation. Sympathy. Empathy. Brooding. Cynicism. Envy.

Heart Meridian

Subscapularis. Heart Meridian. Forgiveness. Compassion. Self-Confidence. Self-Esteem. Self-Worth. Self-Doubt. Insecure. Secure. Anger. Hate. Love.

Small Intestine Meridian

Quadriceps. Small Intestine Meridian. Joy. Shock. Sorrow. Sadness. Internalization. Unappreciated. Nervousness. Overexcited. Discouraged. Assimilation. Nourishing. Hurting.

Abdominal muscles. Small Intestine Meridian. Joy. Shock. Sorrow. Sadness. Internalization. Unappreciated. Nervousness. Overexcited. Discouraged. Assimilation. Nourishing. Hurting.

Bladder Meridian

Peroneus. Bladder Meridian. Fear. Anxiety. Peace. Dread. Terror. Panic. Resoluteness. Frustration. Impatience. Inner direction. Confidence. Inadequacy. Courage.

Sacrospinalis/Erector Spinae Muscles. Bladder Meridian. Fear. Anxiety. Peace. Dread. Terror. Panic. Resoluteness. Frustration. Impatience. Inner direction. Confidence. Inadequacy. Courage.

Tibialis Anterior. Bladder Meridian. Fear. Anxiety. Peace. Dread. Terror. Panic. Resoluteness. Frustration. Impatience. Inner direction. Confidence. Inadequacy. Courage.

Tibialis Posterior. Bladder Meridian. Fear. Anxiety. Peace. Dread. Terror. Panic. Resoluteness. Frustration. Impatience. Inner direction. Confidence. Inadequacy. Courage.

Kidney Meridian

Psoas. Kidney Meridian. Fear. Anxiety. Phobia. Sexual insecurity. Creative insecurity. Superstition. Paranoia. Cautious. Careless. Reckless. Indecisive. Loyal.

Upper Trapezius. Kidney Meridian. Fear. Anxiety. Phobia. Sexual insecurity. Creative insecurity. Superstition. Paranoia. Cautious. Careless. Reckless. Indecisive. Loyal.

Iliacus. Kidney Meridian. Fear. Anxiety. Phobia. Sexual insecurity. Creative insecurity. Superstition. Paranoia. Cautious. Careless. Reckless. Indecisive. Loyal.

Circulation-Sex Meridian

Gluteus Medius. Circulation-Sex Meridian. Gloomy. Hysteria. Relaxation. Stubbornness. Renounce the past. Tranquility. Responsibility. Generosity. Jealousy. Remorse. Calm.

Adductors. Circulation-Sex Meridian. Gloomy. Hysteria. Relaxation. Stubbornness. Renounce the past. Tranquility. Responsibility. Generosity. Jealousy. Remorse. Calm.

Piriformis. Circulation-Sex Meridian. Gloomy. Hysteria. Relaxation. Stubbornness. Renounce the past. Tranquility. Responsibility. Generosity. Jealousy. Remorse. Calm.

Gluteus Maximus. Circulation-Sex Meridian. Gloomy. Hysteria. Relaxation. Stubbornness. Renounce the past. Tranquility. Responsibility. Generosity. Jealousy. Remorse. Calm.

Triple Warmer Meridian

Teres Minor. Triple Warmer Meridian. Elation. Despair. Despondent. Lightness. Heaviness. Loneliness. Humiliated. Hopeless. Serving. Balance. Buoyancy. Solitude.

Sartorius. Triple Warmer Meridian. Elation. Despair. Despondent. Lightness. Heaviness. Loneliness. Humiliated. Hopeless. Serving. Balance. Buoyancy. Solitude.

Gracilis. Triple Warmer Meridian. Elation. Despair. Despondent. Lightness. Heaviness. Loneliness. Humiliated. Hopeless. Serving. Balance. Buoyancy. Solitude.

Soleus. Triple Warmer Meridian. Elation. Despair. Despondent. Lightness. Heaviness. Loneliness. Humiliated. Hopeless. Serving. Balance. Buoyancy. Solitude.

Gastrocnemius. Triple Warmer Meridian. Elation. Despair. Despondent. Lightness. Heaviness. Loneliness. Humiliated. Hopeless. Serving. Balance. Buoyancy. Solitude.

Gallbladder Meridian

Anterior Deltoid. Gallbladder Meridian. Love. Anger. Rage. Wrath. Self-righteous indignation. Forbearance. Motivation. Assertiveness. Boredom. Helpless. Impotent. Passive. Humble. Choice making. Proud.

Popliteus. Gallbladder Meridian. Love. Anger. Rage. Wrath. Self-righteous indignation. Forbearance. Motivation. Assertiveness. Boredom. Helpless. Impotent. Passive. Humble. Choice making. Proud.

Liver Meridian

Pectoralis Major. Liver Meridian. Anger. Rage. Wrath. Distressed. Vengefulness. Resentment. Self-righteous indignation. Transformation. Responsibility. Unhappiness. Happiness. Irritability. Hostility. Content. Bitter.

Rhomboids. Liver Meridian. Anger. Rage. Wrath. Distressed. Vengefulness. Resentment. Self-righteous indignation. Transformation. Responsibility. Unhappiness. Happiness. Irritability. Hostility. Content. Bitter.

Lung Meridian

Serratus Anterior. Lung Meridian. Cheerful. Depressed. False pride. Haughty. Humility. Modesty. Openness. Scorn. Disdain. Intolerance. Prejudice. Contempt. Regret.

Coracobrachialis. Lung Meridian. Cheerful. Depressed. False pride. Haughty. Humility. Modesty. Openness. Scorn. Disdain. Intolerance. Prejudice. Contempt. Regret.

Deltoids. Lung Meridian. Cheerful. Depressed. False pride. Haughty. Humility. Modesty. Openness. Scorn. Disdain. Intolerance. Prejudice. Contempt. Regret.

Diaphragm. Lung Meridian. Cheerful. Depressed. False pride. Haughty. Humility. Modesty. Openness. Scorn. Disdain. Intolerance. Prejudice. Contempt. Regret.

Large Intestine Meridian

Fascia Lata. Large Intestine Meridian. Guilt. Grief. Regret. Release. Self-Worth. Depression. Letting go. Indifference. Unmerciful. Compassion. Sadness. Apathy.

Hamstrings. Large Intestine Meridian. Guilt. Grief. Regret. Release. Self-Worth. Depression. Letting go. Indifference. Unmerciful. Compassion. Sadness. Apathy.

Quadratus Lumborum. Large Intestine Meridian. Guilt. Grief. Regret. Release. Self-Worth. Depression. Letting go. Indifference. Unmerciful. Compassion. Sadness. Apathy.

As you make the connection between your chronic muscle pain and the emotional suffering you've been experiencing, you can begin to contemplate how to unwind some of these patterns.

This may be why your chiropractic adjustments, physical therapy, massage, stretching, regular exercise, steroid injections, food healing, drugs, nutritional supplements or other physical approaches alone have not been making much change in your experience.

Ask what you need to do differently:

- Do you need to feel the emotions more deeply?
- Should you resolve the feelings?
- Should you move the energy that's been stuck in your muscles?
- Something else entirely?

Your body has the wisdom to speak the truth of what you need once you start listening.

What works to overcome pain and suffering? Compassionately understanding your emotional anatomy.

Chapter 5. What Does Your Back Pain Say to You?

"Don't find fault. Find a remedy. Anybody can complain."
- Henry Ford

Your body tries to communicate with you all day long, every day. Are you understanding what you're feeling?

Your body really has only four kinds of problems:

- Blocks
- Congestion
- Resistance
- Interference

How does this relate to what your back pain is saying to you?

A block may show up as lack of energy flow in an acupuncture meridian, in your muscles, in your bones, in your breath. That's why the first thing you want to do on a physical level when you experience back pain is to create length and space.

How do you create length and space?

- Lengthen your spine by standing taller

- Traction your spine
- Stretch your muscles with yoga
- Create space between the vertebrae by bringing your posture into greater alignment.

Congestion may show up as stagnant energy. How does this happen? By sitting. Unfortunately, studies show the average American now sits 9.3 hours per day. Sitting for more than six hours a day makes you up to 40 percent likelier to die within 15 years than someone who sits for fewer than three hours a day – even if you exercise.

How do you break up stagnant chi?

- Take frequent breaks from your chair to get up and move
- Get a standing desk
- Set a timer on your smartphone to remind you to stand up every hour
- Breathe! Lack of oxygen through improper breathing congests your chi

Resistance shows up as disconnection between how you actually feel and what you allow yourself to acknowledge. Simply put, you resist your own emotions.

Back pain may be telling you:

- You feel unsupported in your life
- You carry more responsibility than you're comfortable bearing
- You hold back your true feelings
- You worry about money
- You repress your sexuality
- You feel angry
- You're exhausted but refuse to slow down and rest

How do you stop resisting your emotions? Take a moment to ask yourself: If you weren't afraid to hear, what message would you allow yourself to receive?

Interference comes from outside yourself.

If you think about it, your body knows what's best. Most of us have a cellular memory of what it feels like to be vital, full of energy and radiating happiness.

Interference could be showing up in these ways:

- Poor ergonomics in your chair at work
- Inadequate back support in the car you drive
- Improper cushioning for your neck when you sleep

- One-sided actions (such as a golf swing) that cause your muscles to be tighter on one side
- Overuse of tools such as a hammer, pickaxe or shovel

Years ago I worked with a client who suffered from chronic neck and back pain. She visited her chiropractor every week but continued to struggle until we finally discussed the position of her computer, desk and chair.

Turns out, she habitually sat with her neck twisted to the right and her body contorted to the left so that she could hide from her boss at work.

How do you clear interference?

- Ask a friend to snap a photo of you sitting at your desk at work so you can examine your posture
- Stop schlumping so that your lungs can expand normally to allow yourself to breathe
- Adjust the height of your desk or the position of your chair or body to bring your spine into ideal alignment
- Balance the two sides of your body in a corrective exercise program
- Review the proper use of all tools so that you don't hurt yourself.

What works to overcome pain and suffering? Healing happens when you clear the blocks, congestion, resistance and interference so you can enjoy a healthy body.

Chapter 6. A Medical Intuitive Healer's Guide to Mending a Broken Heart

"Those who have suffered understand suffering and therefore extend a hand."
- Patti Smith

One of the deepest forms of suffering you can ever experience is the heartbreak you feel from the loss of an intimate partner.

On the Holmes and Rahe Stress Scale, divorce and marital separation come in second and third as the most stressful life events right after the death of a spouse, the No. 1 most crushing event that can ever happen to you.

For younger folks, the scale also includes a scientific measurement of the stress caused by the split with a boyfriend or girlfriend, a wretched event no matter when you endure it.

Whether your spouse passes away, you soldier on through a divorce, you haul your stuff away from your lover's apartment or break up with your boyfriend or girlfriend, the complete and utter agony you experience may cause not just emotional torture but also physical distress.

As the late Southern writer and humorist Lewis Grizzard

once put it: "They tore out my heart and stomped that sucker flat."

At any point in a relationship, an energy healer can read the cord connections between you and your loved one. Here's how this works.

When you form an intimate relationship, you form invisible cord connections with your partner. If you want to see for yourself what these cord connections look like, author Barbara Brennan illustrated them beautifully in her book *Hands of Light: A Guide to Healing Through the Human Energy Field.*

Even if you can't see the connections, you can feel when you are deeply connected with someone and also sense the shift when the ties have crumbled.

In addition to your lovers, you form cord connections with your mother, father, brother, sisters and close friends. These connections speak volumes about the depth and breadth of your relationships and how you relate to one another.

1st Chakra connections: At this energy center, you consider each other to be family. You derive identity by being related to each other and sharing financial responsibility. When you are hitched here, you feel you're part of the same tribe.

2nd Chakra connections: At this energy vortex, you feel sexually attracted to each other and draw power from the other person.

3rd Chakra connections: When you relate here, you feel what the other person feels and experience empathy, compassion and caring.

4th Chakra connections: When you truly love another person, you link deeply from your heart to their heart.

5th Chakra connections: When you join here, you have a lot to communicate to each other. You listen well and speak your truth to each other.

6th Chakra connections: When you associate here, you share your visions of the world.

7th Chakra connections: When you connect here, you form a deep spiritual association that may have spanned even more than this lifetime. This includes your karma together and deep life lessons you teach each other.

Whenever you go through the agonizing process of breaking up with another person, these cords gradually split away.

You may have totally disconnected from your partner or vice versa. In contrast, I have had clients divorced from their previous partners for as long as 12 years who have continued to maintain their cord connections.

The problem is that when you keep these old cords, you may experience what I personally describe as "psychic whack." What I mean is that all of a sudden you may feel bad for no apparent reason because you are quite literally picking up on your previous partner's energy.

When you have broken up for good, it's important to cut the cords with your ex-lover so that you can start afresh, unencumbered by the energetic debris of your past relationship.

Failure to cut the cords may prevent you from moving forward wholeheartedly into any new relationship. Or you may discover yourself being pulled back into the drama with your ex even though you know you're no good for each other.

As you cut the cords, speak from your soul to the soul of your previous partner, literally getting off your chest all previously unexpressed words and emotions. The other person doesn't actually have to hear what you say. When you set your intention to communicate soul to soul, the other person will get the message.

Once you have cut the cords and spoken your peace, I then do a karmic healing to complete all spiritual lessons between the two of you. These lessons may occur on the

mind-grid level, your DNA level or the karmic-contract level or from the core of your soul going back through multiple lifetimes.

When you do the energy work to cut your cords and the spiritual work to complete your karma, you don't need to keep going back and reliving the misery. You can move forward in freedom and begin to experience inner peace once again.

Healing your broken heart from the loss of your relationship becomes a crucial step in your recovery. If you don't do it, your heart will remain closed.

When your heart is closed, you are either punishing yourself, protecting yourself or both.

When you keep your heart closed over time, you restrict your life energy. You may feel fatigued and not know why. No amount of rest, exercise, drugs or supplements may help.

You also close yourself off to future love, unconsciously giving up on one of life's greatest joys.

As sorrowful as breakups may be, know that your shattered heart can be healed and you are strong enough to open yourself to love again.

A highly trained energy healer can clear out your heart chakra (and your other chakras), releasing any and all cord connections that remain from previous relationships.

In my professional opinion, the world needs more energy healers who can rebuild heart chakras because heart disease is the No. 1 cause of death for people of all ethnicities in the United States, including African Americans, Hispanics and whites.

Maybe it's not just lousy diet, fatty foods or lack of exercise that hurt your heart. What if you need to let go of the sorrow from past relationships?

Next, you want to clear your self-destructive patterns. It's not uncommon when you go through a breakup to fall into numerous bad habits that adversely affect your mental, emotional and physical health.

The record in my healing practice is more than 400 layers of self-destruct, which I found in a client who had suffered from six forms of cancer.

You may notice you have fallen into self-sabotaging patterns such as drinking too much alcohol, overeating, avoiding socializing and other manifestations of giving up. Once you have stopped this pattern, you can begin to forgive -- a process that blesses you at the deepest levels.

Jesus was asked, "Lord, how many times shall I forgive my brother or sister who sins against me? Up to seven times?"

Jesus answered, "I tell you, not seven times, but seventy-seven times." Matthew 18:21-22

Here are two simple but highly effective forgiveness mantras. You can use both at different times or choose one and repeat it until you feel the energy shift completely between you and your former lover one.

Ho'oponopono, an Ancient Hawaiian Practice of Reconciliation and Forgiveness

I Love You [name of person],
I'm Sorry [name of person],
Please Forgive Me [name of person],
Thank You [name of person].

My Simplified Version of Forgiveness Mantra

I Forgive [name of person],
[name of person] Forgives Me.
I Love [name of person],

[name of person] Loves Me.

As you repeat either or both of these forgiveness mantras, place your hand over your heart. While you're reciting them silently or aloud, you can add the following eye movements to access all parts of your brain:

Eyes Open

eyes up
eyes down
eyes right
eyes left

Eyes Closed

eyes up
eyes down
eyes right
eyes left

How will you know when you're finished with forgiveness? When you can think of the other person and not trigger any negativity, you're done.

To my way of thinking, forgiveness is very much like housecleaning. You may vacuum your house carefully one day only to discover a few days later that more dust has settled and you need to go after it again.

Yes, there are many effective healing methods for your heart. Thank God we live in an age where surgeons can save your life with a heart bypass, nutritionists can change your body chemistry by teaching you how to eat well and you can strengthen your cardiac muscle by working out.

But from my professional experience, I believe it's the failure to overcome the breakups in our lives that causes a gradual restriction of energy to our heart.

It takes tremendous courage to forgive completely but ultimately you can make yourself stronger and perhaps one day be ready to love again.

What works to overcome pain and suffering? Healing happens when you take the time to heal your heart. By practicing unconditional kindness for yourself and all others, you radiate a joy that uplifts everyone around you.

Chapter 7: Why Resolving Long-Term Emotional Stress Is Crucial for Recovery

"We are more often frightened than hurt; and we suffer more from imagination than from reality."
- Lucius Annaeus Seneca

One key to overcoming chronic pain is to resolve the emotions that keep you operating out of your amydalae, *i.e.*, your brain's two tiny "fight, flight or freeze" survival centers.

Over the years, I've worked with countless clients with chronic fatigue syndrome (CFS), fibromyalgia and other multi-system, autoimmune intractable illnesses not easily alleviated by traditional medicine.

Clients have come to me even on oxycontin, one of the strongest narcotics, and I can attest to the fact that no amount of Schedule 2 drugs can accomplish the degree of long-term pain relief you can experience from giving up the survival patterns you hold at the cellular level.

Medical science now corroborates that long-term activation of your amygdalae will cause inflammation in your body leading to chronic pain and depression and that retraining your amygdalae and becoming less emotionally hypersensitive are essential for resolving these illnesses.

Simply put, if you are stuck in survival mode, you will certainly be stuck with chronic physical aches.

What are your amygdalae? Although people often talk about your amygdala (singular), you actually have two amygdalae. These are football-shaped structures located in the temporal lobes on either side of your brain. They are considered to be part of your limbic system, the section of the brain responsible for managing emotions, long-term memory, behavior, motivation and smell.

In my book *Unlimited Energy Now,* I explained that being stuck (or limited) to operating out of your amygdalae -- as opposed to the frontal lobes of your pain -- is a major cause of not only chronic pain but also chronic exhaustion.

I like to keep things simple, so here's the way I explain how your amygdalae operate: When information comes into your brain, the amygdalae act like an airport control tower.

They are located about three-quarters of an inch inside your brain at about the level of your hairline in front of your ears.

If you feel safe, the amygdalae send signals to your frontal lobes so you can think logically and produce your own natural antidepressants and anti-anxiety neurotransmitters. You take in the information and then act from all the wisdom you have gathered throughout your lifetime.

If, on the other hand, the information hits your amygdalae and you feel any sense of alarm, they send signals to the back of your brain -- your reptilian brain -- where you simply fight, flee or freeze.

When you operate out of your reptilian brain, you are in survival mode. Your muscles lock in chronic tension, your inflammatory markers go up, and your breath tightens.

All logic goes out the window. You become unable to access the wisdom of your frontal lobes, and you simply react.

This is known as an amygdala hijack.

You could be a Harvard-trained Ph.D. or have years of experience in natural healing and still find yourself stuck in a high degree of physical and emotional agony.

Which emotions activate your amygdalae? Here's a list from a chart created for kinesiologists by Bruce and Joan Dewe:

- **Surprise:** stupefaction, shock, stunned, startled, astonishment, dumbfounded, amazement, wonder, dazed, awe
- **Disgust:** revulsion, scorn, abhorrence, contempt, disdain
- **Fear:** apprehension, panic, wariness, terror, nervousness, dread, fright, edginess, concern, anxiety, qualm
- **Anger:** irritability, hatred, exasperation, resentment, annoyance, animosity, outrage, hostility, wrath, fury
- **Shame:** chagrin, humiliation, mortification, regret, embarrassment, remorse, guilt, contrition
- **Sadness:** sorrow, melancholy, cheerlessness, self-pity, depression, gloom, grief, loneliness, dejection, despair
- **Love:** acceptance, friendliness, trust, kindness, affinity, devotion, eros, infatuation, adoration, agape
- **Enjoyment:** contentment, delight, happiness, rapture, bliss, amusement, relief, satisfaction, thrill, gratification, pride, sensual pleasure, euphoria, whimsy, ecstasy, mania, joy

Just naming the emotions that throw you into survival mode is a major step forward because it takes you out of the experiencer into the observer state.

Can you observe your emotions instead of being controlled, strangled, overwhelmed or ruled by them? If you suffer from chronic pain, it's very much worth your while to study this list of emotions.

If you are unsure which emotions have you stuck, just ask yourself, "What vibe am I living in today?"

You are a vibrational being. Your heart is electrical. Your brain is electrical.

When you stand up, you are of course vertical, and your electricity creates an energy field perpendicular to your body. New Age people call this your aura.

Other people can feel the energy you give out even if you don't speak about what is bothering you.

All illness or disease -- no matter what label you put on it -- is slowed-down vibration.

As an energy healer, if I put my hands on a hurting area, I may feel heat, congestion or a total block.

True healing occurs when you increase your frequency.

You put yourself in the vicinity of high-vibration energy -- love, beauty, understanding, kindness, forgiveness, fresh air, sunshine and healing foods -- and your frequency shifts.

You may have experienced pain relief simply by walking in the park, giving and receiving hugs, taking a deep breath or saying a heart-felt prayer.

If you are unsure of the emotional patterns that are keeping your chronic pain stuck in place, ask yourself what people are bringing out in you.

If you constantly feel frozen and unable to move forward in your life, you may be experiencing some degree of surprise. Shock is so disempowering it may shut you down completely.

You hold shock in every joint in your body – your feet, ankles, knees, hips, wrists, elbows and neck. So, if you are suffering from constant joint pain, ask yourself if you have experienced shock or surprise.

After the 9/11 terrorist attacks in 2001, I spent an entire month lifting every client who came to me out of shock.

You could witness the impact on the streets of Atlanta as fewer cars than usual were on the road. Life seemed to come to a halt as our entire country processed the destruction and loss of the World Trade Center in New York City.

If you feel contempt and look down on others, you may be suffering from disgust.

If you can't relieve your anxiety, you are stuck in fear.

If other people constantly piss you off and make you endlessly frustrated, you are suffering from chronic anger.

If you can't get over deep embarrassment, you may be suffering from shame.

If you have experienced loss in your life and can't get out of your depression, you may be stuck in sadness.

And finally even deep enjoyment may activate your amygdalae when it borders on mania.

Upon humble reflection, what you may notice is that whatever you think you're experiencing out there – outside in the world – actually comes from inside of you.

Whatever you feel deep inside is what you tend to experience in the world today because you project your emotions everywhere.

That's why learning to release your negativity is an essential life skill for being happy, healthy and pain-free. Once you have humbly acknowledged your emotions, the next key is to move the energy.

Emotions are nothing to fear. They are simply energy in motion -- as long as you keep them in motion.

As an acupuncturist friend of mine, now deceased, once said to me, "There are death, taxes and emotions." All are unavoidable aspects of the human experience. The key is how you handle them.

Failure to keep your emotional energy moving results in stuck energy in the body that any highly trained energy healer can sense.

Ask yourself these questions:

1. On a scale of 0 to 10, with 0 being none, what is the level of tension in your body?
2. On the same scale, what is your pain level today?
3. What can you do right now to release the tension by any amount?

Once you recognize the direct connection between your chronic tension and the interminable pain, you may be motivated to find even the smallest, easiest ways to reduce your internal pressure.

One of the simplest ways to begin retraining your nervous system is to practice yoga, qi gong and breath work. All three modalities allow you to redirect the energy from the survival centers of your brain to your frontal lobes. Through these practices, you learn how to live your life with much less stress and therefore much less pain.

You literally retrain your amygdalae.

You can reduce your tension dramatically and at the same time learn the degree to which you have power over your direct experience.

Even if you can reduce your stress by a mere two percent – and likely more if you practice yoga, qi gong and breath work regularly – you can experience much less pain.

Chapter 8. Choose Not to Suffer

"The storm is not as important as the path it opens up."
- Mark Nepo

If I am going to do a healing to release any common discomfort -- let's say a crick in your neck -- I have to treat your experience of pain and suffering as two separate phenomena. There is the pain itself, and then there is the suffering you choose to experience. I have to release the emotion behind the physical pain, or the energy will simply shift into another area of your body.

Recently, a client received the lab test results for her adrenal gland function. Each of us has two adrenal glands -- one on top of each kidney -- that release adrenalin and cortisol, our stress hormones.

Most people have no clue how much their metabolism, endocrine system, brain chemistry, bones, muscles and even skin and hair have been damaged by their inability or unwillingness to stop the pattern of relentless stress. Most new clients come to me in varying degrees of adrenal burnout, but this particular client won the lottery -- she had virtually no cortisol, a syndrome recognized in traditional medical literature as Addison's disease.

Many people with hypocortisolism would have been lying in bed, disabled by chronic fatigue. My client, however, could function quite well on the surface. She ran a business and took care of her husband and kids. Admittedly, she felt absolutely terrible, which is why she became my client, but she still seemed to be keeping everything up and running.

My client had learned not to complain and focused instead on how much she loves her work, her family and her entire life. She was beginning to turn herself around because she had mastered her inner game.

When we feel annoyed or dismayed and start whining, we set ourselves up to experience more and more suffering.

How can this be?

We keep ourselves stalled and stuck in the same vibrational pattern when we choose to see ourselves, the world and everyone in it as damaged, broken or anything less than how it's all divinely meant to be.

But because we're still human, we all need to sigh every once in a while.

And every so often, it may be helpful to let yourself have a pity party. You could set a timer for say 30 minutes to let out your disappointment. Beat a pillow. Shake your fists at the sky. Kick the garbage can.

Get it all out of your system, and then shift your energy by saying a prayer of heartfelt gratitude for everything you can feel that's actually wonderful.

I have a few treasured friends who can smell my personal pity parties coming a mile away. They smack me down quite helpfully when they see one coming.

You have got to love friends like that.

When I have beginners in yoga class, I like for them to work on plank position, a pose that teaches you how to handle your own body weight. I watch how they handle not just the exercise but also their feelings.

Can you handle the burden of your own weightiness? If not, then lighten up, mentally and physically!

Staying stressed has become a habit for so many people. Is it normal for you to feel constant joint aches, brain fog, weariness, despair, anxiety, and/or heaviness?
If so, then part of you is choosing that experience either consciously or subconsciously. You could very well select another observation point for life. You could choose not to suffer.

To get over your habit of complaining, use these affirmations:

Every day in every way, I am getting better and better.

I choose the best possible thoughts.

I always see the best in myself and others.

Today I choose to experience heaven on earth.

Chapter 9. Give Up Your Payoffs

"Often it's the deepest pain which empowers you to
grow into your highest self."
- Karen Salmansohn

If you've been in physical pain or emotional suffering for
a long period of time, you have to ask yourself if you are
either consciously or unconsciously juicing the payoff.

A "payoff" is often referred to as a secondary gain.
Consciously or unconsciously, you get something out of
staying stuck in your misery.

Simply by releasing the payoff, you can move forward
and step out of your uncomfortable pattern.

If I'm working with a new client who has been unwell for
a lengthy period, one of the first things I do is identify
the payoffs and then do a healing to clear them.

If you don't clear your secondary gains, you can fix your
swollen ankle but then fall down the stairs and hurt your
wrist. You can lose 50 pounds but then contract a
serious disease. And so on.

Trust me, unless and until you root out the payoffs, your
evil inner twin will find a way to keep you miserable.

What are the most common payoffs for remaining fat, sick, hurting, depressed, heartbroken, unhappy, wretched, desperate, troubled, anxious, hopeless, wounded and/or tortured?

- **No responsibility:** If you are sick, you don't have to take out the garbage, get a job, earn a living, get up in the morning or become somebody.

- **Avoid suffering:** Somehow you view staying the way you are as a pathway to avoid the pain of growth.

- **Avoid rejection:** You could be choosing to stay overweight so you can avoid being rejected by members of the opposite sex. You use your excess weight as an excuse to avoid dating.

- **Get taken care of:** This is a biggie. As long as you stay sick, other people have to make your meals, do the chores around the house or support you financially.

- **Superiority:** You are so important and your issues are so special that no one can heal you. You might have to go to a specialist in another country, for God's sake, or find someone with multiple initials behind their name because ordinary solutions just won't work.

- **No commitment:** You don't have to commit yourself to an exercise or eating plan or some other activity requiring discipline to make progress. You can just do whatever you please and stay the way you are.

- **Permission:** Your illness or excess weight gives you permission to make excuses for yourself. You don't have to go to the party, wear a bathing suit, work long hours, or be accountable to other people.

- **Sympathy:** Another biggie. Being sick or overweight may be the only way you know how to get attention.

- **Freedom:** Being sick, you can finally quit your job and do whatever you want to do.

- **Stay independent:** You don't have to listen to the experts. You can just keep doing whatever you want to do, eating whatever you like, and avoiding taking care of yourself because you would rather self-destruct than listen to anybody who knows how to make you feel better.

- **Dependent on others:** You can keep other people at your beck and call because you can't do things for yourself.

- **Guilt:** You can use your illness or excess weight as a way to manipulate other people. They have to come and visit, stay married to you or neglect their own needs because you are so unwell.

- **Control:** Your needs are so specific that you have to control everything about your environment. You decide what goes in the pantry, the lighting, the noise level, etc. It's all about what you need.

- **Victim/Martyr:** Another biggie. You get attention by suffering. You are the victim of other people. You take on everybody's troubles and woes.

- **No decisions:** You don't have to make choices because you are simply too tired to think straight.

- **Apathy:** You can't possibly address the real issues in your life because you are too busy being sick or overweight.

- **Attention:** Any type of attention -- even negative attention -- will do for you.

- **Manipulation:** You use your condition to manipulate other people. You are so unwell their lives must revolve around meeting your needs.

- **Security:** Because you have an incurable whatever, other people and entities, perhaps including even the government's permanent disability program, must take care of you for life.

- **Blame:** You are so sick because someone else has hurt you. It's all the other person's fault. If only this person hadn't been so horrible, you could be living a normal life.

- **Identity:** You are your illness. You are a card-carrying member of the incurable disease support group, and your entire social life revolves around being a member of a sick collection of people.

- **Safety:** It's a lot easier to lie around the house being sick or overweight than it is to go out and take a risk in life.

- **Avoidance of intimacy:** How could you possibly have sex or form a relationship when you feel so bad?

- **Avoidance of listening:** You feel so poorly, you just don't have the energy to listen to other people or care about their issues.

- **Grow up:** Being sick keeps you in a permanent state of infancy. Other people make decisions for you, pay your bills and make long-term plans on your behalf.

You have to ask yourself: Do you honestly want to get well? If the answer is no, then you're juicing the payoffs and won't truly get well until you release them.

Chapter 10. The Healing Power of Self-Compassion

"I think modern medicine has become like a prophet
offering a life free of pain. It is nonsense. The only thing
I know that truly heals people is unconditional love."
- Elisabeth Kubler-Ross

One block that may hold you back from releasing
unpleasant patterns in your life is your relationship with
yourself.

The teeny-weeny habit of finding constant fault with
yourself -- often disguised as a never-ending quest for
self-improvement -- gets in the way of your true healing.

The most healing frequency of all is the vibration of
unconditional love, a love that you'll be happy to learn
requires nothing of anybody, including yourself. You
don't have to be or do anything to experience the benefit
of this frequency. You just have to be in the
neighborhood.

Just as sunshine penetrates the darkness, unconditional
love can softly caress and brush away the inevitable
wounds of life.

One of the easiest ways to begin to practice
unconditional love is through compassion.

What is compassion? It's a quality of your heart. It's more than just empathy.

You may have empathy for others when they lose a spouse, end up in a hospital, fall down and hurt their knee, get fired from their job or end up with the sniffles. In those situations, it's sometimes easy to rationalize that whatever happens to others isn't even really personal -- it's just part of the human experience. Everybody aches sometimes.

Compassion happens when you expand your heart energy. This may occur most often in a nonverbal manner, without your saying or even doing anything.

You can feel your heart, and others can feel it, too. It's as if your heart is radiating a steady energy that warms everyone around you.

What if you could offer the same compassion for yourself? Although we can receive compassion from family, friends, doctors, energy healers and all other members of the helping profession, perhaps the most important person to have this quality of heart for you is you.

That's because you can't really let in all the love that exists for you until you allow yourself to be in a compassionate, loving relationship with your true self.

Here are a few ways you can expand this heart quality to include yourself:

- **Catch yourself in the habit of self-judgment.** When you notice yourself finding fault with who you are, what you look like, how much money you do or do not make, how far you think you have or have not come in your life and all the myriad ways you can measure yourself to some imaginary standard, just stop for a moment. Where did these ideas come from anyway? Mother, father, church, mass media, your friends? Or you simply decided you need to be that way? What if you could simply allow yourself to be you with no labels? Have mercy on yourself and give yourself permission to throw away your old measuring sticks.

- **Soften your expectations.** Even if you truly believe you should be marching forth in some other fashion, what if you could allow yourself to be who you are, where you are in this very moment? By letting go of your preconceived ideas, you allow your true self to emerge from under all your masks. Practice tenderheartedness with yourself. Allow your process to play out rather than forcing or constricting it. Just let yourself be you.

- **Notice how you can love yourself just the way you are now.** You may not be living in your ideal situation with the comfort and ease you would prefer, but being hard on yourself won't make anything better. Can you allow yourself simply to be? Can you accept and welcome the way you are now, recognizing your beauty, strength, tenacity, and perseverance in spite of all that has happened? By letting go of the habit of pushing or shoving yourself in one particular direction, you allow your highest good to show up by grace in perfect timing.

What works to overcome pain and suffering? Healing happens when you hold yourself tenderheartedly in mind, compassionately allowing your humanity and trusting God to guide you to all that is good, blessed and wonderful.

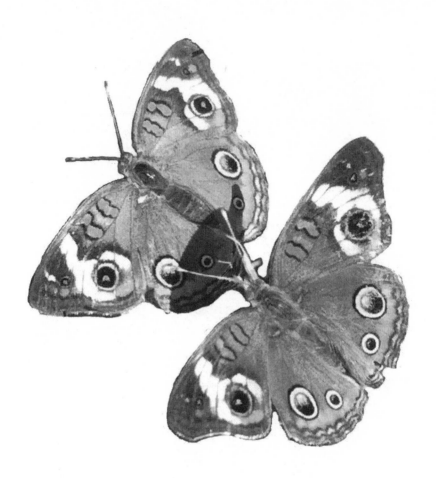

Book V

Your Mental Body

Chapter 1. The Truth Will Set You Free

"The truth will set you free. But not until it is finished
with you."
- David Foster Wallace

Recently a woman came to see me about her back pain.
She had been diagnosed with spondylolisthesis, a very
nasty condition of the spine. It's likely at least one of her
vertebrae was shoved forward out of place, possibly
squeezing her spinal cord or nerve roots.

She was facing surgery and didn't really want to go under
the knife. She had been to see a chiropractor but hadn't
experienced permanent relief and wanted to find natural
ways to get rid of her pain.

I taught her six exercises and in the space of less than 90
minutes she managed to bring her pain level down from
an 8 out of 10 to a 2.

For each exercise, I showed her what to do, then had her
copy what I was doing in her own body. She took
photographs as I demonstrated each exercise correctly. I
also typed out written instructions and explained the
finer points in great detail.

After each exercise, I would have her walk around to
discover the difference in her own body.

From an 8 to a 6, a 6 to a 4, a 4 to a 2 1/2 and then finally she got to a 2.

"You needed me about 40 years ago," I observed.

Her spinal condition was quite severe. I couldn't promise that what I taught her could reverse spondlyolisthesis, but she could feel for herself how she didn't need to suffer from the condition as severely as she had been feeling it.

"Go home and repeat what I taught you, then do it again every day. Twice a day wouldn't be too much."

Pain has a way of getting our attention. The sharpness, its constancy, the experience of suffering drags us out of our present reality into a dimension where we often feel trapped.

We can become so convinced of the reality of pain we come to the conclusion that this is just the way it is.

Life sucks. Or does it?

Do you really want to belong to the largest cult in the world -- DIFFICULT -- or would you rather your life be easy?

Is it true that your only option is to be in pain or take

drugs and go under the knife with surgery?

Is it true that depression, anxiety, and hopelessness have to be a part of your journey or could you feel differently?

As you contemplate your options -- whether you have been diagnosed with spondylolisthesis or some other dreadful ailment -- you can get out of your own way by asking yourself the following questions.

1. What would I be experiencing right now if I did not have this condition?

A few days after her initial visit, my client with spondylolisthesis came back for a follow-up. I had taught her one exercise that required no equipment -- only a corner of a wall.

"I know you're going to think this is pathetic but I can't find a corner in my house," she explained to me.

"I have so much stuff everywhere. I know what you are going to say to me," she continued.

"Just deal with it. Move stuff out of the way. Make it happen."

Would you be willing to move the furniture in your house, in your mind, in your soul, or would you rather continue to experience torment?

"You could go outside," I pointed out to her helpfully.

"Find a wall outside your house. Put down a mat or a towel and practice your exercise in the fresh air."

If you have a solution -- if you already know what you could do to encounter even a little less discomfort -- you have to ask yourself what you would be experiencing if you didn't have this condition.

Are you using your condition as an excuse? What are you really avoiding?

2. Am I willing to accept this condition?

Many people put up with low-level aches, depression, anxiety, and annoyances. When your pain is a 4 out of 10, you may just make a habit of accepting it.

In my opinion, it's actually helpful when your discomfort level reaches a 7, 8, 9 or even a 10 because your focus is finally so intense that you may force yourself to find a solution.

Do you really want to put up with this?
Have you convinced yourself that your life is a vale of sorrow?

Are you ready to become fed up with yourself and your situation and deal with it?

3. If someone somewhere could wave a magic wand, would I be willing to let it go?

Not that I am a believer in magical thinking, but you have to ask yourself: If a great magician could wave away your anguish, could you or would you actually just be done with it?

If you can honestly answer yes, then you may be ready.

If you instinctively admit you kind of like the agony, then the first place you really need to work is between your ears, examining whether you're juicing the entire experience for the payoffs.

4. Has anyone else anywhere in the world been able to relieve themselves of this condition?

Medical miracles do exist. Natural healing can do wonders. I myself have healed more clients with chronic back pain than I can even count.

One woman burst into tears during our first visit because she had struggled for two years despite undergoing physical therapy and massage and could hardly believe all her misery was gone in less than an hour.

If you can find anyone anywhere who has overcome the very same adversity, then hope exists for you too.

5. What would I need to be, do, have or think to experience complete and utter relief?

You cannot be the same person with anguish as you will be when you free yourself from this torture. To become a pain-free person, you have to be, do, have or think totally differently.

Ask yourself:

- What do I need to be?
- What do I need to do?
- What do I need to have?
- What do I need to think?

For example, my client with spondlyosthesis might have to:
- Be consistent with her daily exercises. Even if she cannot relieve the condition permanently, consistency can help her to choose a totally different experience.
- Have a clean corner.
- Think she is actually worth taking care of.

What works to overcome pain and suffering? Healing happens when you allow self-inquiry to reveal the truth about what you need to be, do, have or think to experience complete relief from your discomfort.

Chapter 2. The Story You Tell Yourself
Creates Your Chemistry

"Nothing ever goes away until it has taught us what we
need to know."
- Pema Chodron

Recently, I conducted medical intuitive readings for two
women who had experienced severe trauma. One
woman's son had been murdered two years previously.
Another had experienced bullying at work. Although the
hectoring happened some 20 years ago, she recalled the
humiliation as if it had just occurred yesterday.

Your story either kills you or heals you.

Every time you tell a story inside your head – even if you
don't speak it out loud to anybody else – you recreate the
same chemistry as the day the event happened. Maybe it
doesn't happen with the same intensity, but on a cellular
level you deepen the injury's grooves.

You don't just recall the anguish. You don't just see the
picture of what happened inside your head. Instead, you
trigger and reignite the neurotransmitters in your brain
today that made you as shocked, devastated and
unhappy as the day it first happened.

For example, if I say, "Think about biting into a lemon,"

you experience a certain chemistry in both your mouth and your brain.

It may have been years since you actually bit into a lemon, but when you think about it you are creating the exact same experience on a cellular level.

As I explained this fact to the woman who had been bullied, she recognized the impact on her thought patterns immediately. "In essence I'm making it happen – making it deeper and deeper," she said.

Your story can keep you stuck if you don't change it. That is why you may experience constant physical pain and emotional suffering without relief despite receiving help and support from the most well-meaning traditional or alternative therapists, the best surgeons, the kindest ministers and the most loving family.

You're doing yourself no favors every time you go back in your mind and relive the traumatic experience, however innocently you may return to it.

The woman whose son had been murdered had visited countless healers and therapists. Her family kept advising her to let it go, but she didn't know how.

She kept seeking answers and hoping for justice that never came.

The killers were never caught. Her son could not return. She cried even as she told me the full story. Her loss was as awful as ever.

I told her that what I saw in my medical intuitive reading was that the only thing that would heal her completely was to write a book, to let her soul pour forth through pen and paper.

She had etched and stored the pain of losing her son so deeply inside her, it wasn't just in any one particular organ. It was in every cell of her body.

"Another medium I consulted told me the exact same thing," she said.

"Well," I replied, "then it must be true."

About an hour or two after our session, she received an email from a writing coach inviting her to a free lecture to learn how to write a book. She forwarded the email to me. Spirit had spoken to her three times and she got the message!

If you've accidentally stepped on a land mine, don't continue to blow yourself up day after day. Often the truth is that the things happening to us are so awful we must be careful not to relive them inside our minds.

You may not see yourself choosing that outcome, such as stepping on the land mine day after day, but in truth that's what you're doing if you get stuck reliving your story.

Sometimes we catch ourselves watching the experience in our minds to try to figure it out, to search for understanding about how or why it occurred. As you do this, though, realize you may in fact be re-injuring yourself and making it difficult or impossible to let go of depression, anxiety, physical pain and emotional suffering.

How do you stop the trauma inside your head?

How do you cease making yourself sick?

You can tell your story a better way.

Here's how I recommend you rewrite your story without changing one iota of fact.

1. **Write your story as positively as you can.** You must resist the temptation to change any facts because your ego mind as well as your soul know what really happened. Don't tell yourself any lies. Just relate the story as positively as possible.

2. **Reread.** As you reread your own story, notice your emotional reaction. If you experience any negativity, notice where in the story you start to cry or feel angry.

3. **Rewrite it again.** Keep rewriting your story until you experience NO negativity at all in the retelling of it. You can set your story aside for a few days and keep coming back to it. Over time, your soul will reveal the better way to remember it.

If your trauma feels so real you can't put it into words, draw a picture. Then draw it again as you would like to remember what happened.

I developed this approach from personal experience.

When I went through a divorce in 2010, I recognized the impact of what was happening and decided I didn't want my recollections to make me sick.

So I would write the story in my journal. After a while, I would return and reread and eventually rewrite.

It took me a few months, but today I can recall what happened and not relive any of the pain. I know for a fact that I went through a divorce, I know it was one of the most difficult things that ever happened in my life, but when I ponder further, I don't relive the anguish.

I can recall my divorce with the same emotional impact as if I had said, "I went to the grocery yesterday." Completely neutral – that's your goal.

Nobody told me to do this. I just figured it out.

I noticed how I felt every time I thought of all the bad things that had happened. I would look in the mirror and see the tension in my face. I didn't want to stay that way.

A side effect of this process is that my ex-husband and I are now actually very good friends. He comes over for dinner, we go to the movies. We can be in each other's presence and I don't relive the suffering. We have experienced complete forgiveness.

Today I'm even healthier than I was seven years ago and I give part of the credit to the way I handled my story. Your inner peace is there for your uncovering.

How can you rewrite the story you tell yourself truthfully so that you can get to inner peace?

1. **Each story may have a villain but there will also be a hero.** For example, Batman may fight multiple bad guys but he's the hero of his own story. Maybe you're the hero of your story. Maybe you survived. Perhaps other

people stepped in to help you out of the goodness of their hearts and became heroes in your eyes. If you look, you can feel the loving kindness all around you.

2. **Find the blessings**. Because we live in a friendly universe, the truth is that it's all one energy. It's all God and it's all good. In your mind look to see how your soul grew, examine the insights you received, and witness the blessings that have been showered upon you.

3. **Receive the lessons.** Maybe the worst thing that ever happened to you taught you how to forgive. It's my experience that what we think of as total trauma on an ego level often becomes our greatest teacher on the soul level. The people we consider our worst enemies are often our best friends spiritually speaking.

4. **Pray to God for help.** Often we get so stuck in our tales of misery or woe that we have trouble lifting the veil. Ask God to show you the truth about what happened – not the truth as your ego perceives it, but the divine wisdom. What it looks like to me as a medical intuitive healer is you peel away

layers of what you call reality. As you do this, you shed your own pain, no drugs, surgery or natural healing remedies required.

What works to overcome pain and suffering? Healing happens when you rewrite the story that has caused you to feel sick and suffer.

Chapter 3. Think Like a Rich and Healthy Person

"You are the universe expressing itself as a human for a
little while."
- Eckhart Tolle

After 24 years of empowering other people to be
healthier and happier, I have come to the conclusion
that rich and healthy people think alike.

Over the years I have coached many millionaires and
paid attention to how they think.

"The key to business is low overhead," one
multimillionaire once told me.

I listened. Soon thereafter, I moved my business to my
home, a choice I have never regretted, especially as I
listened to friends and colleagues sweat over their
expensive rents for fancy offices.

Working in this simple location, I've empowered
countless clients to overcome every kind of extreme
health challenge so completely you couldn't possibly tell
they ever had a problem in the first place.

Yes, I help people with natural healing, the most
effective exercises, the healthiest ways to eat and the

fastest-acting stress management techniques, but there's more to it than that.

I empower you to think differently because you can't think the way you thought when you were poor or sick and expect to experience anything else.

Here's how this works.

Are there things you need to do to be wealthy or healthy?

No doubt.

Are there better techniques, smarter financial vehicles, wiser investment advisers, more experienced personal trainers, more advanced nutritional products?

Of course.

At the end of the day, it's all about your mindset.

The greatest predictor of your wealth and your health is the way you think. When you think thoughts over and over again, they become your beliefs. Your beliefs establish the inner landscape for your choices.

When you think the same thoughts and make the same choices day in and day out, you either become wealthier and healthier or poorer and sicker.

Let me give you a few examples from my own life.

Even though I have never made an outlandish income, I have no debt. My house is paid for. My nine-year-old Prius is paid for.

Of course this didn't happen overnight. It took years to pay off my home loan but I made it a goal. I paid off my car as quickly as I could.

When I charge anything on my credit cards, I go home and pay off the charge through my online banking system within 24 hours.

I don't buy anything I can't afford.

Not to say I don't live well – anybody who has seen my wardrobe or the contents of my refrigerator can attest to that.

The secret of financial success is to live within your means.

By remaining debt-free, I keep my energy in present time because I'm not worrying about my financial future or regretting past mistakes about poor spending choices.

Even though I'm currently 58 years old, I have no pain.

If and when I injure myself, I deal with it immediately.

I visit a chiropractor or a craniosacral therapist, practice yoga to work out my sore muscles, enjoy a hot bath to relax or take whatever steps are necessary to eliminate the ache.

I exercise every day and take vitamins, herbs and homeopathic remedies. I maintain ongoing coaching appointments and regularly consult with a good friend who is a naturopath because you should never be foolish enough to be your own doctor.

Yes, this costs money but I save by being drug-free and therefore not having to pay for doctor visits, lab tests or expensive monthly prescriptions.

Because I've been taking care of my health for decades, not only do I not look my age but I'm building up a reservoir of personal chi that will ward off degenerative diseases that break down countless other people. Chiefly, we're talking about diabetes, adrenal burnout, osteoporosis, anxiety and depression, hormone imbalances, high blood pressure and high cholesterol, arthritis and many other common illnesses too numerous to mention.

Just as I don't build up a backlog of debt, I don't build up a backlog of physical discomfort or emotional distress.

In short, when stress arises, I deal with it right then and there, just like I pay off all credit charges within 24 hours.

Many times when I am practicing therapeutic yoga with a client who has been suffering back pain, knee pain, hip pain, shoulder pain or literally any other pain, I find myself thinking a simple thought:

"This is not that hard."

Of course it's not hard for me because I've taught fitness, nutrition and natural healing for 24 years, topping out as a master wellness coach with about 48,000 hours of practice.

I like to show you the easiest way to do anything. That's because if I show you the easiest way, I know you are more likely to do it and keep doing it.

And if you keep it up more than likely you're going to become one of the healthiest, happiest people in your circle of friends and family.

Many of my clients who have become ill or hurting have

simply let their physical well-being slide – often for decades. A good example popped up during a recent call from a prospective client in England.

"I had a problem during one of my pregnancies," the caller related to me.

She said she is currently in her early 60s. Her problematic pregnancy happened more than 30 years ago and she hasn't felt well since.

During not just one but three decades after the problem first surfaced, she may have been able to rewrite her story and shift the way she felt by simply choosing to place a higher priority on her health. "To feel better you have to value the way you feel," I advised her.

Here's how rich and healthy people think alike:

1. Rich people value their money.

2. Healthy people value their health.

3. Rich and healthy people seek out the smartest people they can find to continue to take their money and their health to the next level.

4. No matter their income level, rich people live within their means.

5. Healthy people don't overeat, get overly stressed or waste their time or energy.

6. If they have to charge something on their credit cards or take out a mortgage or loan to buy a house or start a business, rich people place a priority on paying off the debt as quickly as possible.

7. If and when they become sick or injured, healthy people do whatever it takes to deal with their physical, mental and emotional issues immediately.

8. Rich people build their wealth by saving money even before they think they might need it.

9. Healthy people build their health by exercising daily, taking natural healing remedies and managing their stress before they ever get sick.

10. Rich and healthy people see taking care of their own well being as a gift not only to themselves but as a legacy to their families and everybody around them, becoming a literal wellspring for others.

If you want to know what you really think about money or health, simply listen to your inner dialogue. What do you say to yourself when nobody else is around?

Do you say:

- It's hard for me to make any money.
- It's difficult for me to lose weight.
- I can't get out of debt.
- I can't get out of misery.
- I can't lose weight (if you think you can, you can).

Or do you say:

- I've got a great plan and I'm working my plan.
- I enjoy being debt-free.
- I'm so thankful to feel great.
- I choose to be the best I can be.
- I feel younger than my age.
- I love my life.

If you notice your thought processes are keeping you stuck, change the problem where it actually starts – between your ears.

When you change the way you feel and think you can change your external results.

Why not feel fabulous?

It's less exhausting.

Why not look fabulous?

It's more fun.

Why not be financially free?

It's less stressful.

Why not be radiantly healthy?

You'll have the energy to live life the way you really want.

When I was growing up, my father used to say to me, "You only go around once."

Make it count by choosing to think like a rich and healthy person.

Chapter 4. Affirmations for Healing

"I do not fix problems. I fix my thinking. Then problems fix themselves."
- Louise Hay

You can direct your mind to uplift your personal energy despite immense suffering.

Here are some of my favorite affirmations you can say to yourself at times when your hurt may feel unbearable.

EVERY HAND THAT TOUCHES MY BODY IS A HEALING HAND.

I AM DIVINELY GUIDED TO THE PEOPLE, PLACES, METHODS AND PRACTICES THAT PROVIDE TRUE RELIEF FOR ME ON ALL LEVELS NOW.

GOD IS GOOD ALL THE TIME AND I NOW GIVE MY TORMENT TO GOD.

THANK YOU GOD FOR BLESSING ME WITH EXCELLENT HEALTH THIS DAY AND FOREVER MORE.

I LET GO AND LET GOD HEAL ME.

I TRUST THE PROCESS OF MY HEALING AND ALLOW DIVINE WISDOM TO LEAD ME TO ALL THAT IS ACTUALLY HELPFUL.

I NOW JOYFULLY RELEASE THE EMOTIONS AND THOUGHT PATTERNS THAT HAVE CAUSED ME TO SUFFER.

INNER PEACE FLOWS THROUGH EVERY CELL OF MY BODY AND BRINGS RADIANT HEALTH TO ME ON ALL LEVELS NOW.

I FEEL MY DIVINE CONNECTION AND ALLOW THE SPIRITUAL ENERGY TO BRING ME THE RELIEF I NEED AND WANT.

I KNOW MY GOD TAKES CARE OF ME EVEN IN THE MOMENTS OF MY GREATEST SUFFERING. I CALL IN MY ANGELS, SPIRITUAL GUIDES AND DIVINE GUIDANCE TO LIFT ME UP.

I INVOKE THE LIGHT OF THE CHRIST WITHIN, I AM A CLEAR AND PERFECT CHANNEL, LOVE AND LIGHT ARE MY GUIDES. I FORGIVE ALL PAST EXPERIENCE, I AM FREE.

I NOW GIVE UP THE RIGHT TO HOLD ON TO ANGER, GRIEF, RESENTMENT, FEAR, REVENGE, INNER TURMOIL AND BITTERNESS

AND ALLOW GOD TO FLOOD MY BEING WITH UNCONDITIONAL LOVE FOR MYSELF AND ALL LIVING BEINGS NOW.

THANK YOU FOR THIS HEALING IT IS DONE BY GRACE IN DIVINE TIMING.

I SEE MYSELF AS WHOLE AND COMPLETE JUST AS I AM NOW.

THANK YOU GOD FOR BLESSING ME ALL THE DAYS OF MY LIFE.

MY HEART AND MIND ARE FULL OF GRATITUDE.

NOTHING COMES IN AND NOTHING GOES OUT EXCEPT UNCONDITIONAL LOVE.

I AM RADIANTLY HEALTHY.

MY RADIANT INNER BEING EXPRESSES ITSELF OUTWARDLY IN THE FORM OF EXCELLENT HEALTH.

Place your hand over your heart as you repeat these affirmations.

Visualize yourself as whole, healthy, complete, happy, smiling and full of the life energy you need to fulfill your soul's purpose. Record these affirmations in your own voice on your smart phone and listen to them repeatedly throughout the day.

Speak your healing into existence and it will come!

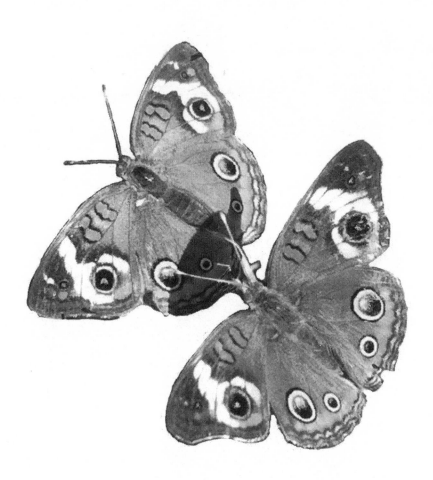

Book VI

Your Spiritual Body

Chapter 1. What Beauty Will Come from Your Pain?

"Behind every beautiful thing there's some kind of pain."
- Bob Dylan

She was young-ish, in her early 30s, and studying to become a psychologist.

She told me her choice was between working with me to relieve the constant discomfort of her scoliosis or spending more than $3,000 to purchase a back brace that she would wear every day.

Knowing that she was on two antidepressants as well as oxycontin, a.k.a. hillbilly heroin, I chose to tread carefully.

Just by the fact that she was on so much medication, I understood that she had been having a hard time handling life's struggles.

At our first session I simply taught her how to stand, sit and lie down with the best possible posture to avoid aggravating her back.

We didn't do a single exercise. I didn't offer any healing work. I just taught her how to cope with the basic positions her body would assume throughout the day to avoid aggravating her condition.

She came back two days later to report that whatever we had done with her posture had touched off a wave of spasms so severe she had chosen to increase her dosage of oxycontin.

Given that most people not only feel better when they stand, sit and sleep with good posture, I knew what I was really dealing with was not her spinal distortion but her own inability to experience life outside her pain body.

"Let's do a healing for you to be willing to get out of pain," I recommended.

She listened. We discussed the payoffs she had been receiving for staying in torment. I helped her see that she had been consciously and unconsciously juicing the experience.

After that visit, she never returned.

Sometimes our aches speak so loud that no other voices can be heard outside our own mind. We can even lose touch with the truest internal guidance system of our own souls.

As a person who was studying psychology to assist others

with the travails of life, she herself was just beginning to understand.

We can never judge another person's path.

Every hero's journey starts out by battling a demon.

It is possible that by now this very same woman has found a way to free herself from the discomfort of scoliosis, rid herself of her dependency on oxycontin and be happy without antidepressants.

In my 24 years of work in holistic healing, I have helped countless clients become pain-free despite scoliosis, get off even heavy dependency on oxycontin and learn how to be happy enough that even their doctors agree they no longer need psychiatric medication.

As a recoverer, a survivor, a person who has triumphed over herself, my former client with scoliosis might offer tremendous hope for those still stuck in their suffering. Sometimes the depth of your own sinking predicts the height of your personal rebound.

As you contemplate the ache within, one of the questions you can ask is, "What can I make of this that will make the whole thing worth it?"

As a medical intuitive healer, sometimes just for fun when I'm out enjoying a public lecture, I will observe the person speaking and read their body, mind and soul.

I'll never forget listening to a very influential Atlanta preacher.

As I watched him speak, I recognized his brain profile was transposed, which meant that the usual left brain functions were happening in his right hemisphere and vice versa. I saw that in his earlier years, he had fallen into the drug culture.

Somehow he had seen the light and had come so far. CEOs of Atlanta's biggest corporations often sought him out for spiritual direction.

His compassion was as much of an asset as his brilliant mind.

You may discover the beginning of your journey as the choice between facing your issues or merely living in a back brace to tolerate them.

Where will your journey lead you?

As you discover the strength inside yourself to face your affliction, you create a vision of possibilities for all those left behind in the struggle.

What works to overcome pain and suffering? Healing happens when you see the beauty of your journey, even if you haven't yet reached the end of your story.

Chapter 2. Sometimes All You Have to Give Is Love

"Love has power in it. At the end, it wins over all miseries."
- Debasish Mridha

There are times when no matter how hard you wish or try, you truly cannot alleviate another person's torment. Hope as you might, try as you might, their torture exists beyond the reach of your personal influence.

Recently my mother came to Atlanta for my niece's high school graduation. We all sat through the two-hour ceremony. Only upon coming back to the house for a meal afterwards did my mother mention that she felt anything other than wonderful.

"Will you help me?" she asked.

"Of course," I responded.

I knew she wanted me to give her yoga exercises to alleviate the shooting pangs radiating from her neck and upper back down into her arm.

So we went down to the basement of the house where my niece lives and I made do with the few pieces of equipment I could gather - a yoga mat, a strap, a foam roller, a chair, the back of a couch and the walls of the room.

Even as we worked through the gentle exercises, my mother did not complain. But I could tell the ache was more than she could bear.

She asked to stop before I was ready to finish.

I knew I could not force anything.

The next day, a Sunday, I called my mother to hear how she was doing. It was 2 p.m.

I was surprised to learn she had already made the four and a half hour drive to Savannah.

"I got up at 6 a.m. to drive home," my mother admitted. This time she began relaying a little more of the truth about her hurt.

"Please go to the emergency room," I begged her.

I called my brother, the doctor, and within minutes he and I were off the phone. Within the hour my mother was waiting at an orthopedic emergency center.

The doctors prescribed pain medication.

I called the next day to check on her progress: no relief. And the next day: not any better.

And the next.

I texted my mother's physical therapist. I begged my mother to make an appointment for acupuncture (you always have to make do with the therapies a person is willing to accept) but the next available time slot wasn't until the following week.

Finally a doctor prescribed even stronger medication.

The physical therapist worked with my mother two days in a row at the end of the week.

"Are you any better than you were last Saturday?"
"Not really," she admitted.

If I had it all my way, my mother would have seen a non-force chiropractor for an adjustment, the acupuncturist she had previously visited, a Reiki master for energy healing, a neuromuscular therapist for release of her trigger points and a yoga therapist for correction of her kyphosis. She also would have been taking natural anti-inflammatories rather than prescription drugs.

But it wasn't my journey. It was her path and I could still love her all the way through.

Eventually her MRI showed she had a herniated disc in her neck. My mother ended up integrating massage into her recovery plan and agreed to attend physical therapy three days a week. She acknowledged her body needed more care than she had been giving it.

Meanwhile, as I was reaching out to my mother day by day, I was texting back and forth with a client whose ailing mother had just been rushed to the ICU.

"This is my worst nightmare," my client wrote.

I wrote a prayer for my client and her mother and hit send in the text box.

My client's mother passed away shortly afterward.

"I am completely heartbroken," my client wrote back. "I don't really know what to think. She is the first person to show me unconditional love. A daughter is a daughter forever and she will always be with me. I'm grateful for the years that I had with her and I know she will be with me.

"Mommy, I love you more than words could ever describe."

I sent my client a photograph of a butterfly.

This beautiful butterfly posed for me in August 2015 when I was at a yoga retreat. I probably took at least 50 photos of him.

"I'm sending you this image to remind you that you are surrounded by love and light even in the moment of your greatest loss. I'm so sorry you are suffering. Please hold this image in mind and let this beautiful butterfly comfort you."

I was winding down after hearing of my client's loss when I looked at my Twitter feed and discovered there had been yet another terrorist attack in London.

I reached out through Facebook to an old friend I hadn't talked with in a while.

The last time she and I had communicated was after a previous London terror attack a few months earlier.

"Are you OK?" I asked. "Just heard of the news from London – sending YOU lots of love and light!"

She confirmed that she was indeed safe but had recently been diagnosed with edema in her bone marrow. She had been hobbling around on crutches and was hoping to take time off work to recover from emotional exhaustion after her father had passed away.

"Processing all the trauma from my childhood," my dear friend confided. "Working through everything and just working out how to give up work for a while as I can recover!!"

I encouraged my friend to give me a ring over Skype when she felt like talking. And then she was off to bed.

That night I got down on my knees and prayed for everyone in the city of London. I prayed for the police who were protecting the city. I prayed for the ambulance drivers and the nurses and doctors at the hospitals. I prayed that everyone who had been injured would be healed. I prayed for everyone who died. I said words of forgiveness for the terrorists. Soon enough I ran out of words to pray and got up off my knees.

Sometimes all you have to give is love.

And that can feel like nothing and yet it can in fact be everything.

What works to overcome pain and suffering? Healing happens whenever you send the vibration of unconditional love.

Chapter 3. Call on Your Power Animals

"We don't heal in isolation, but in community."
- S. Kelley Harrell

Years ago, I performed a medical intuitive reading for a woman in Kenya who was a big cat researcher. Both she and her husband had spent years in the wild filming, studying and advocating for the lions, tigers and leopards not just in Africa but all over Asia.

Unexpectedly, she had fallen ill. A mutual friend recommended she call me for a healing.

She was out of reach of modern medicine and in a country where even the usual natural healing remedies I would advise her to take could not be obtained.

I recommended that she call on her power animals, the big cats, for healing.

Often in life it seems like we've been cut off from the people, medicines and resources that might most easily provide relief.

On such occasions, we must turn to the spirit world, knowing and experiencing that we are never truly alone, never cut off from divine assistance and always looked after at the deepest levels.

Whether you know them or not, you have power animals in the spirit world to whom you can turn to for assistance.

I first learned of my own mother snow leopard when visiting a shaman.

Nothing was really wrong with me at the time, but I was curious what a shaman would advise me to do. He told me about the snow leopard who had been walking with me my entire life.

Soon thereafter, I began seeing the big cat in my meditations. She is strong, graceful and silent.

Snow leopards are among the rarest of the big cats, so when the leopard and lion researcher called for my assistance I knew exactly where to send her for help.

Explorers can search for years before seeing their first snow leopard. These long-tailed cats exist in remote regions in the Himalayas, wandering high up the slopes and blending in with the rocky mountain sides.

On a spiritual level, snow leopards give you the power to leap over any obstacle.

Their long tails give them a strong sense of balance.

They live close to God in thin air, rarely coming into contact with humans.

I have called on my mother snow leopard many times, visualizing myself riding on her soft strong back as together we leap over any obstacle.

As the years passed, a second snow leopard appeared in my meditations, this one a little cub.

While my mother snow leopard has gravitas, my baby snow leopard always wants to pounce and play.

Soon after I met my baby snow leopard in meditation, my soul met my hawk, flying high above, giving me a sense of the big picture, and a hummingbird capable of blessing me with endless joy.

About a year ago a dragonfly came into my psyche, helping me to break illusions and adapt easily to change. When you are ready, your soul can make contact with your power animals for comfort, relief and healing.

Power Animal Meditation

Step One. Come to a comfortable position, either lying or sitting down.

Step Two. Close your eyes and say a prayer.

HEAVENLY FATHER,

THANK YOU FOR MY LIFE, FOR ALL THE ANGELS AND SPIRITUAL GUIDES WHO HAVE BEEN WALKING WITH ME ALL THE DAYS OF MY LIFE.

IF IT IS THY WILL, PLEASE REVEAL MY POWER ANIMAL TO ME NOW.

CALL FORTH THE SWEET SPIRIT OF MY POWER ANIMAL INTO MY INNER VISION THAT I MAY SEE AND EXPERIENCE THE WISDOM, COMFORT AND BLESSINGS OF THIS DIVINE BEING.

ALLOW MY POWER ANIMAL TO HEAL ME AT THE GREATEST DEPTHS, TRANSFORMING MY BEING FOR THE HIGHEST GOOD, RELEASING AND TRANSMUTING ALL THAT HAS KEPT ME FROM EXPERIENCING THE BLESSINGS OF LIFE ON EARTH.

THANK YOU GOD, THANK YOU GOD, THANK YOU GOD.
AMEN.

Step Three. After you say your prayer, allow your mind to fall silent.

In the inner landscape, notice the power animal who appears out of the air, prancing through the forest, swimming through the sea, crawling, prowling or leaping into your inner vision.

Look deeply into the eyes of your power animal and allow the contact to be made. Listen at your soul level. You may hear, see, feel or know the message your power animal has for you today.

Spend all the time you want in your inner landscape with your power animal. Allow yourself to experience this special soul friendship.

When you are ready, silently thank your power animal, knowing you are accompanied at all times by the most magnificent, loving, caring being you have ever met.

Open your eyes now and go about your day feeling centered in your inner truth.

Chapter 4. Raise Your Vibration Past the Suffering

"Find a place inside where there's joy, and the joy will burn out the pain."
- Joseph Campbell

One of the simplest ways to move past suffering is to ask yourself just one question: "How can I raise my vibration?"

This is the precise question I ask on my client's behalf whenever I do healing work.

What will most efficiently heal your body, mind and spirit?

What will lift you beyond the physical ache, past your emotional misery, and into an entirely new realm of existence?

It's a simple way of thinking, but this one question often produces the most profound results.

All illness – no matter whether you stub your toe, battle cancer or are blowing your nose constantly with a common cold – is simply slowed-down vibration.

Even if you have never thought of it that way, you can

instinctively understand what I'm talking about.

Just think of the last time you went to a nursing home.

The energy there feels so slow, so congested, you can't wait to leave. Five minutes there feels like an eternity.

And nothing will exhaust you like a week with the flu. You felt so good just a few days ago, now you can hardly lift your head off a pillow.

You can shift this slowed-down energy simply by increasing your frequency.

Heal yourself anytime, anywhere, by giving yourself permission to raise your vibration.

You'll know you're there because you experience a spark of joy, even just for a moment, for a full breath, for five minutes, for an hour.

What can you do to raise your vibration past the suffering?

- Watch a funny movie
- Laugh at a good joke
- Call a friend
- Practice deep breathing exercises
- Smell a flower

- Hug a child
- Walk in the fresh air
- Pet a puppy
- Tickle a baby
- Listen to the purr of a kitten
- Dance to your favorite tunes
- Play a game
- Write a poem
- Sing a song
- Sit in silence
- Show up at church, the synagogue, your mosque
- Pray
- Meditate
- Attend the opera, a play, a live concert
- Visit a botanical garden
- Watch a live football or baseball game
- Say "I'm sorry" and really mean it
- Forgive everyone who has ever hurt you
- Stroll down the beach
- Sit beside a lake

This is not just a matter of distracting yourself from the misery, it's a way to shift your internal state.

And if you can't do something different right now or

place yourself in the vicinity of more uplifting energy, you can use your very powerful mind to call upon the wisdom of your soul.

By letting go and trusting God, you can connect to an answer outside the realm of your current understanding. Here's a simple meditation you can do anytime, anywhere, to call on the precise frequency you need to balance your body, mind and spirit.

Step One. Sit in a comfortable position.

Step Two. Turn your palms upward in the receptive position.

Step Three. Close your eyes and say a prayer:

HEAVENLY FATHER, PLEASE BLESS ME WITH THE PRECISE FREQUENCY I NEED IN THIS MOMENT TO HEAL MY BODY, MIND AND SPIRIT. PLEASE ALLOW THIS ENERGY TO BE INTEGRATED ALL THE WAY DOWN TO THE CELLULAR LEVEL. THANK YOU GOD, THANK YOU GOD, THANK YOU GOD. AMEN.

Step Four. Sit in silence and feel what's happening. Notice the shift as you enjoy the peace.
Healing can happen in an instant when you allow yourself space to experience something different.

Chapter 5. What Are You Transforming Through Your Pain?

"The world breaks everyone and afterward many are
strong at the broken places."
- Ernest Hemingway

Years ago I went to the dentist for what I thought would
be a routine cleaning.

"You need caps on two of your teeth," the receptionist
informed me when I went to pay.

"If you come back tomorrow we'll give you 10 percent
off."

Thinking that I might save a little money by facing up to
the issue immediately, I rearranged my schedule and
came back the very next day, only to have the nerves in
my face damaged to such an extent that I ended up with
a four-month case of trigeminal neuralgia, also known as
"the suicide disease," because 25 percent of sufferers
commit suicide.

I remember walking into a health food store and muscle
testing myself among the homeopathic remedies.

"For when your teeth hurt so bad you feel like
screaming," the label read.

Oh, that would be the one!

Immediately after the dental procedure, I wasn't sure why even a slight breeze next to the right side of my face would set off a wave of shooting, throbbing and burning spasms the likes of which I had never experienced.

My brother, a doctor, was the one who diagnosed my condition.

Trigeminal neuralgia is often considered the most agonizing condition in the medical literature, reportedly worse than childbirth or limb amputation.

Your trigeminal nerve is a paired cranial nerve that has three major branches: the ophthalmic nerve, the maxillary nerve, and the mandibular nerve.

When this nerve plexus gets irritated, daily activities such as chewing, talking, brushing your teeth or touching your face can set off an ache that may last between a few seconds to countless hours.

I can remember I had paid a $5,000 to attend a very intense, week-long workshop in New York on anatomy and physiology.

I can't recall anything I learned. All I could think about was going home to see the dentist and get relief.

Unable to escape the agony, I experimented with meditations where I simply directed my mind deeper into the experience. I hoped to dissolve my suffering by accepting it as fully as I could.

But the truth is I was so miserable I couldn't think straight.

Finally I consulted my mentor in healing.

"What is this about?" I remember asking.

"You are dropping all your genetic programming on all levels all at once," my healer concluded.

"No wonder this hurts so bad!" I responded.

It turns out that my father and his mother, my paternal grandmother whom I adored so much, had also suffered from trigeminal neuralgia.

I had been so aggressive about my personal growth work that the wave of energy I had unleashed had surged through my nervous system and was now releasing through my face.

Not soon enough I had not one but two root canal surgeries.

During the first root canal operation, the surgeon gave me five shots of Novocain, and I could still feel the torture as he drilled away into my gums.

The agony finally ended after my second root canal. The procedure was so expensive I figured I must have paid to put the surgeon's children through summer camp.

Despite the cost, I felt like a different person. Deep inside I felt free and more at peace with myself than ever before.

When your adversity tries to get the better of you, you would do well to ask yourself, "What am I transforming?"

What has been welling up inside you, stirring below the surface, that you are ready to release?

Even if you can't put your finger on it, can you transmute yourself into a whole new dimension?

Can you let go of all you have learned, all you have been born into and all you ever known?

What works to overcome pain and suffering? Healing happens when you give yourself permission to release excruciating patterns all the way down to your DNA level.

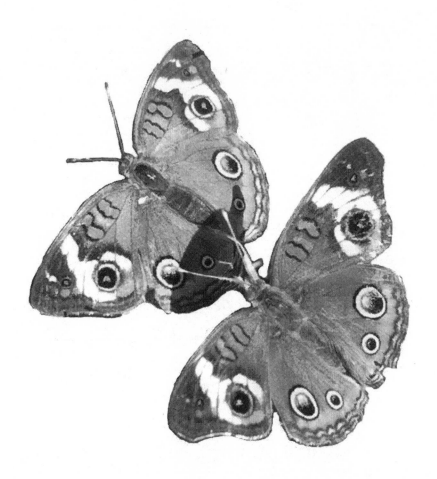

Conclusion

Chapter 1. Remember When You Felt Really, Really Good

"I am better off healed than I ever was unbroken."
- Beth Moore

Just as your cells hold memories of trauma, your body also remembers wholeness – feeling relaxed, happy, easy, comfortable and pain-free.

You remember walking on the beach, the wind blowing in your air.

You remember your first kiss.

You remember a warm hug.

You remember petting your dog, your kitty cat.

You remember the comfort of a hot bath and a cup of tea.

You remember what it feels like to hold hands with someone you love.

You remember looking up at the blue sky, taking a deep breath, seeing the wonder of the stars at night, enjoying the silence.

When I am doing a medical intuitive reading, I often ask how and when your agony started:

- Whether your pain began on the physical, energetic, emotional, mental or spiritual level.

- The age or ages when this pattern started.

- Any other relevant information about how you got triggered.

Just because you hurt now doesn't mean you have to feel that way forever.

Why do I know this is true?

Because your kinesthetic memory is your longest-term memory.

Even if you feel terrible in this moment, more than likely your cells know how to operate in a healthy, harmonious manner.

If I am practicing energy healing, one of the things I typically say to your body is, "Show me radiant health."

You hold this cellular memory of perfect health.

Even if you were born with deformities or deficiencies,

you belong to the human race. Collectively we humans hold a deep understanding of well-being.

Even if you doubt the possibility, you can ask your body to recreate this state of inner harmony.

As we conclude, I would like to leave you with a special prayer.

Chapter 2. Prayer for My Reader

"Don't waste your pain; use it to help others."
- Rick Warren

HEAVENLY FATHER,

THANK YOU FOR THE GIFT OF THIS BOOK. THANK YOU FOR ALL THE INSIGHTS, WHISPERS FROM THE SPIRIT WORLD, AHA MOMENTS AND DEEP SOUL ACCEPTANCES.

I SAY A SPECIAL PRAYER NOW FOR MY DEAR READER.

PLEASE BLESS THIS READER WITH HEALTH, HAPPINESS, KINDNESS, GOODNESS, TOLERANCE AND SELF - CONTROL.

PLEASE SURROUND THIS READER WITH THE WHITE LIGHT OF PROTECTION, THE BLUE LIGHT OF HEALING AND THE GOLDEN LIGHT OF TRANSFORMATION.

IF IT IS THY WILL, PLEASE EMPOWER THIS DEAR READER TO CALL FORTH THE CELLULAR EXPERIENCE OF RADIANT HEALTH AND TO RECREATE THAT VITALITY NOW ALL THE WAY INSIDE AND OUT,

OUTSIDE AND IN, BLESSING THIS DEAR READER WITH RELIEF, WHOLENESS AND JOY.

I ASK THAT THIS BE DONE IN THE NAME OF JESUS CHRIST.

THANK YOU GOD, THANK YOU GOD, THANK YOU GOD.
AMEN.

Appendix: Pain-Free Exercises

"Practice means to perform, over and over again in the face of obstacles, some act of vision, of faith, of desire. Practice is a means of inviting the perfection desired."
- Martha Graham

After teaching yoga for 21 years, I have come up with a list of the 41 exercises I recommend most often for therapeutic purposes. These are the movements I teach my clients to overcome back pain, hip pain, neck pain, shoulder pain, knee pain and exhaustion.

As you practice the exercises, please follow these principles:

1. Use the power of your mind to visualize yourself practicing each exercise before you start. Even if an exercise is outside the range of what you can currently accomplish, you'll receive tremendous benefits by seeing yourself doing it in your mind's eye.

2. Keep your movement 100 percent comfortable. No strain, no discomfort.

3. Keep your range of motion within what your body will easily allow. No pushing.

4. Practice relaxing your whole body, not just the muscles you happen to be working.

5. Breathe deeply. Send loving, compassionate energy to any parts of your body that aren't feeling well.

6. Once you have finished your pain-free exercises, lie down and rest to allow your nervous system to integrate the changes you have made.

7. If you are unsure whether any exercise is safe for your body at this time, please consult an exercise professional.

List of the Pain-Free Exercises

1. Posture Exercise 1 -- Chest Stretch with Strap

2. Posture Exercise 2 -- Overhead Lat Stretch

3. Posture Exercise 3 -- Overhead Letter Y

4. Posture Exercise 4 -- Chest Stretch in Front

5. Posture Exercise 5 -- Perfect Posture

6. Seated Posture

7. Don Tigny Mobilization

8. Wide Leg Forward Fold

9. Cat Cow

10. Hamstring Stretch

11. Supported Fish Over Yoga Eggs

12. One Leg Against the Wall Pose

13. Knee Exercise with a Roll

14. Knee Exercise with Block and Strap

15. Supported Backbend Over Bolster

16. Supported Forward Fold Over Bolster

17. Child's Pose Over Bolster

18. Supported Wide Leg Forward Bend

1. Posture Exercise 1 -- Chest Stretch with Strap

Directions:
- Stand with your feet directly underneath your hip bones. Make sure your feet are pointed straight ahead.
- Bring a yoga strap behind you with your hands hip-width apart.
- Wrap your hands around the yoga strap.
- Keep your wrists straight. Lift up evenly and stretch your chest.
- Breathe!
- Hold one minute.

Benefits:
- Brings your spine into alignment.
- Stretches your chest.
- Allows you to breathe more deeply.

Caution:
- Make sure you don't flex your wrists.
- Make sure your feet are pointed straight ahead.
- Be sure to breathe deeply and relax!

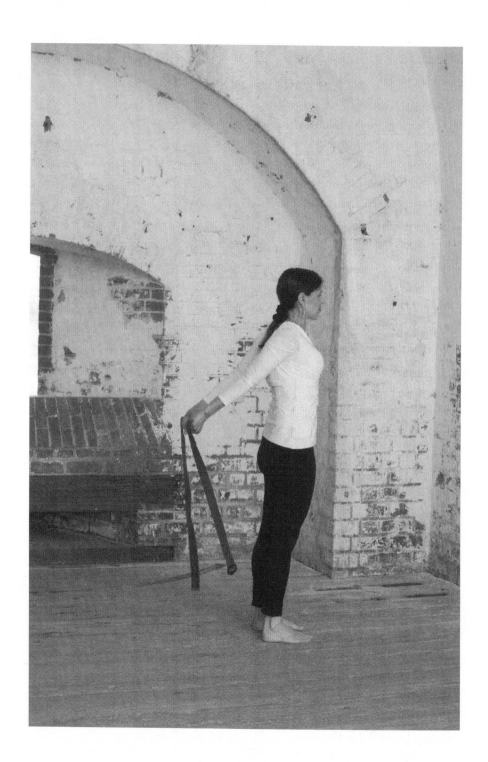

2. Posture Exercise 2 -- Overhead Lat Stretch

Directions:
- Stand with your feet directly underneath your hip bones. Make sure your feet are pointed straight ahead.
- Bring a yoga strap overhead with your hands hip-width apart.
- Wrap your hands around the yoga strap.
- Keep your wrists straight. Pull horizontally to the left and right as if you were pulling the strap apart.
- Breathe!
- Hold one minute.

Benefits:
- Brings your spine into alignment.
- Stretches your latissimus dorsi muscles, the largest muscles in your back as well as your shoulders.
- Increases oxygen flow to your lungs.

Caution:
- Make sure you don't flex your wrists.
- Make sure your feet are pointed straight ahead.
- Keep your arms as straight as possible.
- If you can't bring your arms fully over your head, do your best but don't arch your back.
- Be sure to breathe deeply and relax!

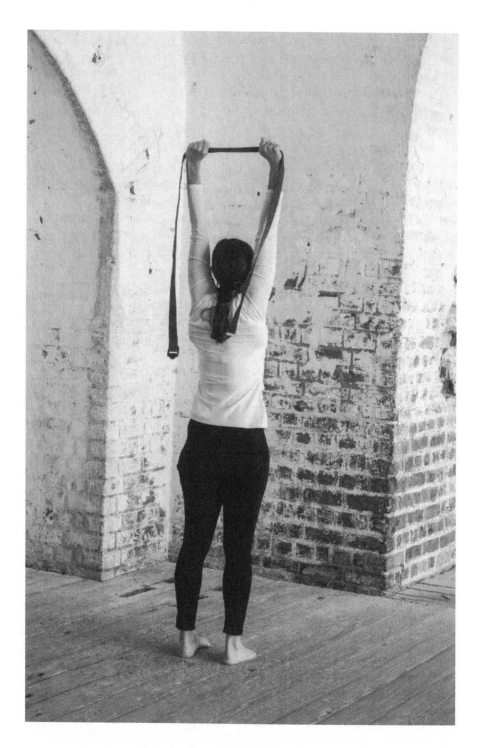

3. Posture Exercise 3 -- Overhead Letter Y

Directions:
- Stand with your feet directly underneath your hip bones. Make sure your feet are pointed straight ahead.
- Bring a yoga strap overhead and make the letter Y.
- Wrap your hands around the yoga strap.
- Keep your wrists straight. Pull horizontally to the left and right as if you were pulling the strap apart.
- Breathe!
- Hold one minute.

Benefits:
- Brings your spine into alignment.
- Stretches your latissimus dorsi muscles, the largest muscles in your back as well as your shoulders.
- Increases oxygen flow to your lungs.

Caution:
- Make sure you don't flex your wrists.
- Make sure your feet are pointed straight ahead.
- Keep your arms as straight as possible.
- If you can't bring your arms fully over your head, do your best but don't arch your back.
- Be sure to breathe deeply and relax!

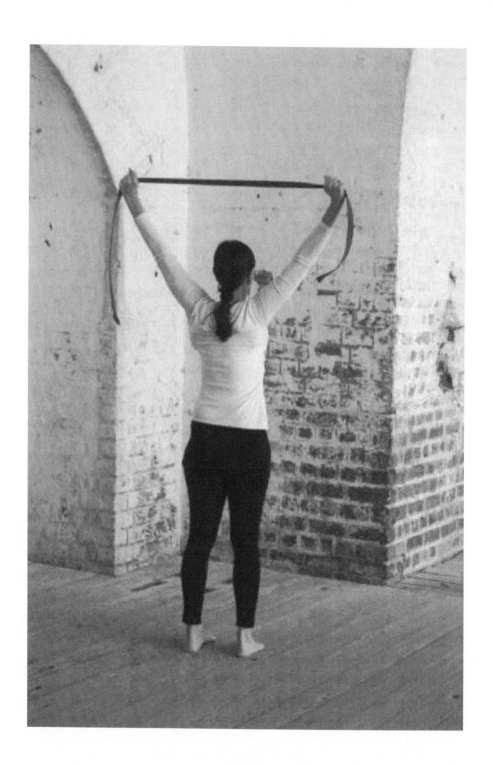

4. Posture Exercise 4 -- Chest Stretch in Front

Directions:
- Stand with your feet directly underneath your hip bones. Make sure your feet are pointed straight ahead.
- Bring a yoga strap in front of your body as wide as your hips.
- Wrap your hands around the yoga strap.
- Keep your wrists straight. Pull horizontally to the left and right as if you were pulling the strap apart.
- Breathe deeply as you practice bringing your whole posture into better alignment.
- Hold one minute.

Benefits:
- Brings your spine into alignment.
- Increases oxygen flow to your lungs.

Caution:
- Make sure you don't flex your wrists.
- Make sure your feet are pointed straight ahead.
- Keep your arms as straight as possible.
- Be sure to breathe deeply and relax!

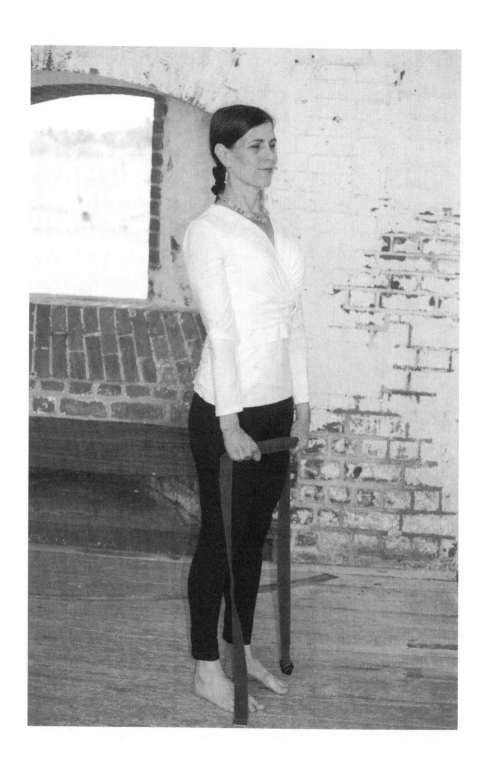

5. Posture Exercise 5 -- Perfect Posture

Directions:
- Put a yoga block or book between your feet.
- Hug the block or book with your feet, pulling your inner groins back toward the center of your body.
- From two inches below your belly button, lift the pit of your abdomen toward the crown of your head.
- Lift and spread your chest.
- Press the back of your shoulders behind you into an imaginary wall.
- Pull your head into alignment over the center of your chest.
- Let your arms hang gently to the side.
- Breathe and relax.
- Hold one minute, then remove the block or book and practice standing straight.

Benefits:
- Brings your spine into alignment.
- Increases oxygen flow to your lungs.
- Trains your body awareness. Notice how your little aches and pains go away just by standing up straight.
- This is the basic posture from which you will practice all your other exercises.

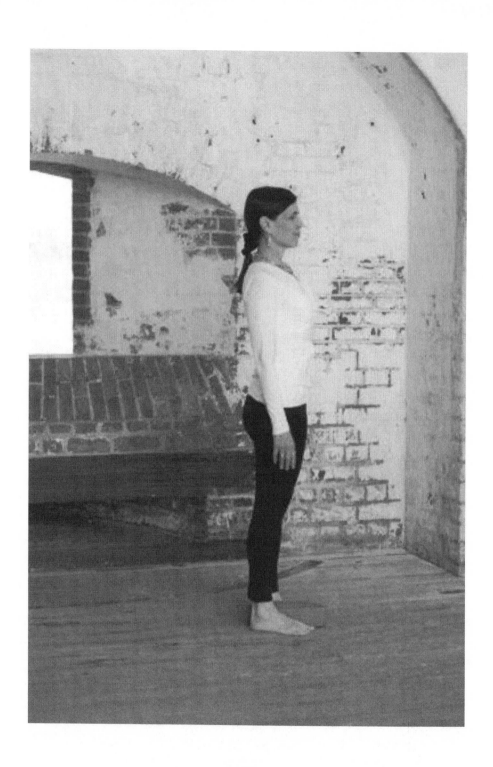

6. Seated Posture

Directions:
- Sit in a chair with your legs forming a 90-degree angle.
- Bring your feet straight ahead and hip-width apart.
- Pull the flesh out from underneath your sit bones.
- Tilt your hip bones gently forward, giving yourself a 30- to 35-degree curve in your lower back.
- From two inches below your belly button, lift the pit of your abdomen toward the crown of your head.
- Lift and spread your chest.
- Press the back of your shoulders behind you into an imaginary wall.
- Breathe deeply as you practice bringing your whole posture into better alignment.
- Hold one minute.

Benefits:
- Brings your spine into alignment.
- Increases oxygen flow to your lungs.
- Trains your body awareness. Notice how your little aches and pains go away just by sitting up straight.
- This is the basic posture from which you will practice all your other exercises.

Caution:
- Make sure you don't collapse your lower back by rolling your hip bones backward.
- Make sure you don't schlump forward into a C position.

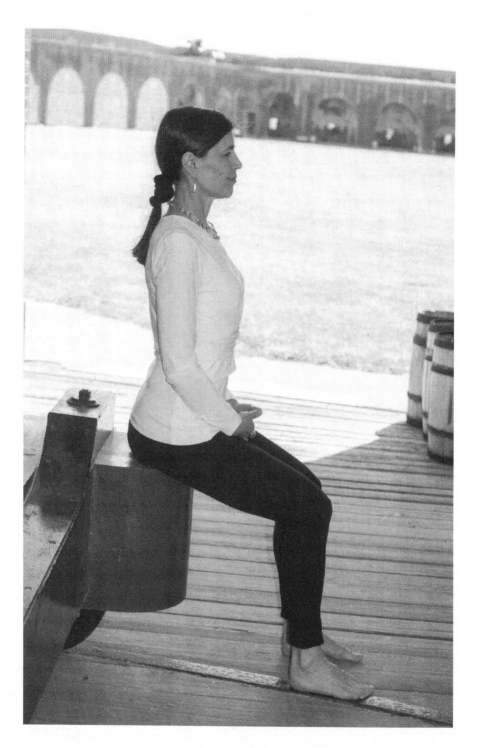

7. Don Tigny Mobilization

Directions:
- Lie on your back with your knees bent, feet hip-width apart.
- Pull your heels toward your buttocks.
- Straighten your left leg with your left foot aiming straight up to the ceiling, setting your hip bone properly in the socket.
- Gently inhale and slowly press your right knee forward, lifting your right hip off the floor about one-fourth inch.
- Exhale as you lower your right hip back onto the floor.
- Inhale as you lift, exhale as you lower.
- Continue one minute before repeating the exercise on the other side.

Benefits:
- Unlocks your sacroiliac joint.
- Relieves low back pain.
- Relaxes your spine.

Caution:
- Move slowly and gently, making this a small movement to unlock your lower back.
- Make sure your feet are straight.
- Be sure to breathe deeply and relax!

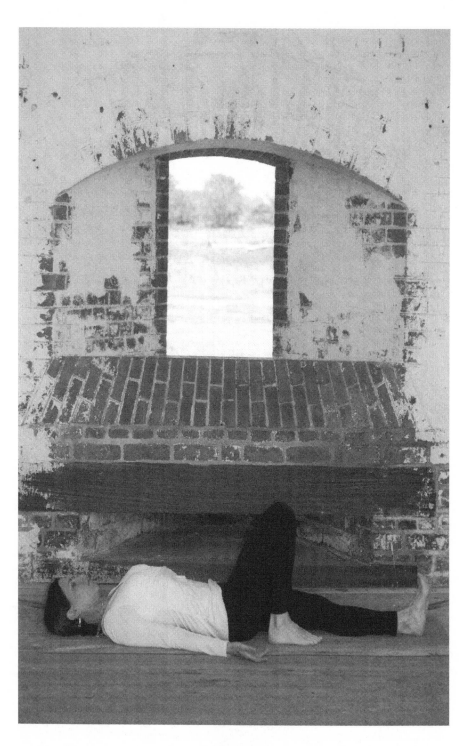

8. Wide Leg Forward Fold

Directions:
- Stand in front of a bed, chair or table.
- Bring your feet wide apart -- so wide that if you had your arms straight out from your body your ankles would be directly under your wrists.
- Turn your feet in as if you were pigeon-toed.
- Press down on the outside edge of your legs as you pull upward on the inside edge of your legs.
- Put your thumbs in your groins and fold at the hips, placing both hands on the bed, chair or table in front of you.
- Tilt your tailbone upward as you pull your belly toward your spine.
- Keep your arms as straight as possible.
- Hold one minute as you lengthen your spine.

Benefits:
- Unlocks your sacroiliac joint.
- Relieves back pain.
- Relaxes your spine.
- Creates space between your vertebrae to traction your spine gently.
- Brings your spine into alignment.

Caution:
- Be sure to breathe deeply and relax!

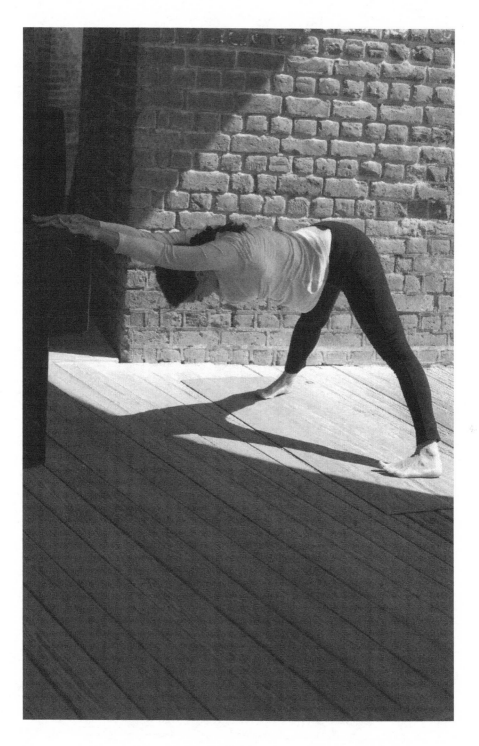

9. Cat Cow

Directions:
- Get down on your hands and knees.
- Spread your knees and hands as wide as your shoulders.
- Keep your arms as straight as possible.
- Keep your wrist crease straight and spread your fingers.
- As you inhale, tilt your tailbone up and gently lift your head.
- As you exhale, round your entire spine, pressing your tailbone forward and tucking your chin to your chest.
- Move with your breath, inhaling as you arch and exhaling as you round, for one minute as you bring flexibility to your spine.

Benefits:
- Unlocks your sacroiliac joint.
- Relieves back pain.
- Relaxes your spine.
- Creates space between your vertebrae to lengthen your spine gently.
- Brings your spine into alignment.

Caution:
- Be sure to breathe deeply and relax!

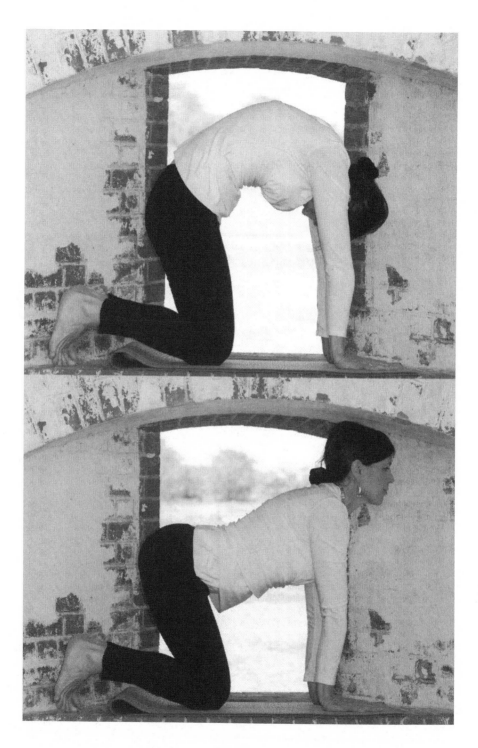

10. Hamstring Stretch

Directions:
- Lie on your back and bend both knees.
- Put a yoga strap on the ball of your right foot.
- Straighten your right leg as much as possible while you gently pull toward a 90-degree angle.
- Straighten your left leg out on the floor and be sure to point your left toes straight up to the ceiling to set the left hip bone in the socket properly.
- Draw from your right kneecap toward your right hip.
- Contract your quadriceps in the front of your right thigh to increase the stretch in the hamstrings in the back of your right thigh.
- Hold one minute, then repeat on the other leg.

Benefits:
- Stretches your hamstrings.
- Relieves back and hip pain.
- Relaxes your spine.
- Improves your posture.

Caution:
- Be sure to breathe deeply and relax!

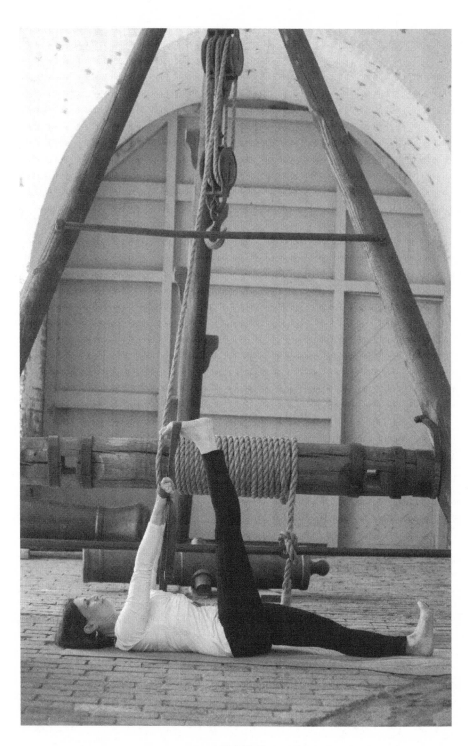

11. Supported Fish Over Yoga Eggs

Directions:
- Put two yoga eggs on the floor leaving a 2- to 3-inch space for the vertebrae of your spine.
- Put a third yoga egg at the top to serve as a pillow for your head. If you have extreme forward head posture, turn the yoga egg on its side, i.e. curved side up, or add a second yoga egg to your pillow.
- Sit on the floor with your back lined up to your yoga eggs.
- Lie over the yoga eggs beginning at the lower edge of your ribs.
- Bring your feet as wide as your yoga mat.
- Roll your shoulders open by turning your palms up to the ceiling.
- Relax in place for seven minutes.

Benefits:
- Relieves back, neck and shoulder pain.
- Relaxes your spine.
- Improves your posture.
- Restores your energy.

Caution:
- Make sure the yoga eggs line up with your ribs.
- Make sure your feet are wide apart.

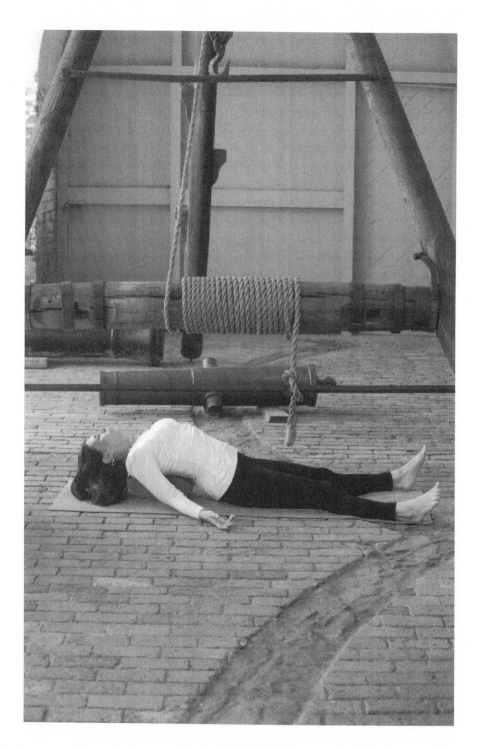

12. One Leg Against the Wall Pose

Directions:
- Find a corner of a room.
- Sit next to the corner and bring your hips onto the wall.
- Hoist your left leg upward at a 90-degree angle straight up the wall.
- Bring your right leg at a 90-degree angle to hug the edge of the corner.
- Keep your legs as straight as possible.
- Drive your left heel gently into the wall.
- Draw from your left kneecap toward your left hip to accelerate the stretch in your left hamstring.
- Relax for five minutes, then repeat on the other side.

Benefits:
- Relieves back and hip pain.
- Relaxes your spine.
- Improves your posture.
- Restores your energy.
- Clears your stress hormones and balances your nervous system.
- Gives your heart a rest.
- This is the easiest way to stretch tight hamstrings!

Caution:
- Make sure you relax and breathe.
- Keep your feet straight.

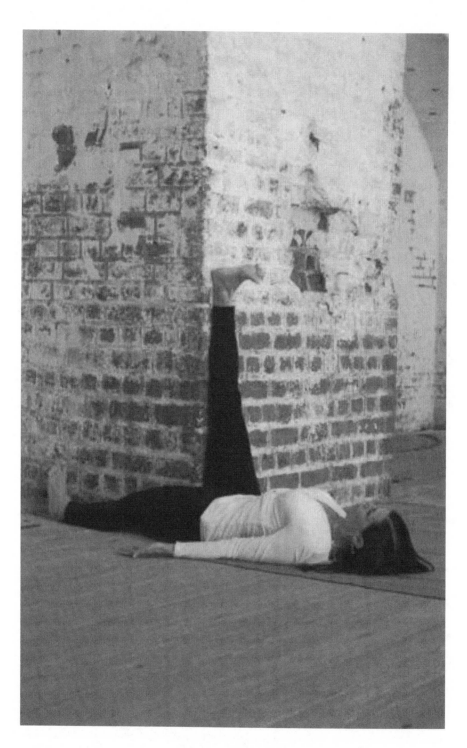

13. Knee Exercise with a Roll

Directions:
- Roll up a yoga mat halfway or roll up a blanket to a thickness of three to four inches.
- Sit on the floor with your right knee bent and your left leg straight.
- Place the rolled-up yoga mat or blanket above the back of your right knee.
- Gently press the back of your right knee into the roll, contracting the quadriceps on the front of your right thigh.
- Contract for a count of three, then release.
- Repeat one minute, then switch to your other leg.

Benefits:
- Relieves knee pain.
- Strengthens your quadricep muscles on the front of your thighs.

Caution:
- Make sure you relax and breathe.
- Keep your feet straight.

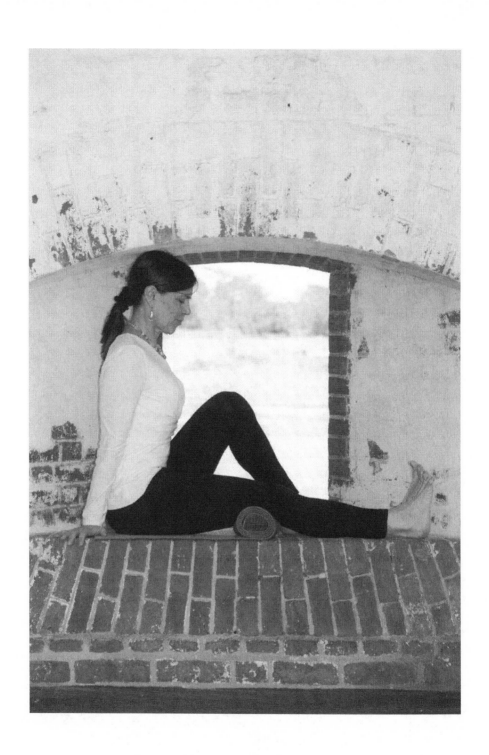

14. Knee Exercise with Block and Strap

Directions:
- Sit on the floor with a yoga block, yoga egg or book.
- Place the yoga block, egg or book between your knees.
- Take a yoga strap and make a belted loop.
- Put the loop around your gastrocnemius muscles-- the rounded muscles at the top of your calves.
- Tighten the belt.
- Press horizontally to the right and left as if you are trying to split the yoga strap.
- Meanwhile, draw from your kneecaps toward your hips.
- Draw from the outer knee toward your hips.
- Contract, hold and push for one minute, then switch to your other leg.

Benefits:
- Relieves knee pain.
- Strengthens your quadricep muscles on the front of your thighs.

Caution:
- Make sure you relax and breathe.
- Keep your feet straight.

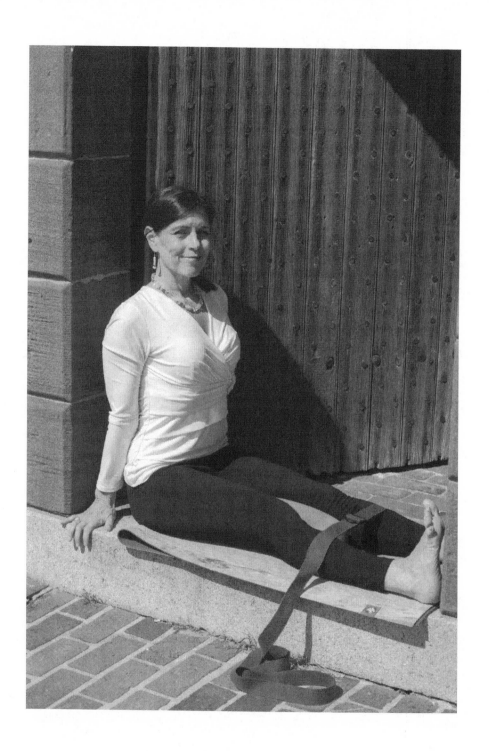

15. Supported Backbend Over Bolster

Directions:
- Place a yoga bolster on top of your yoga mat.
- Sit in front of your yoga bolster.
- Gently lie back with your ribs on the bolster.
- Bring your legs as wide as your yoga mat.
- Lengthen your arms to your sides.
- Turn your palms up to the ceiling to roll your shoulders open.
- If your neck hurts, put a pillow under your head or roll up a blanket to support your head and neck.
- Relax in place for five minutes.

Benefits:
- Relieves back pain.
- Restores your energy.
- Balances your nervous system.
- Releases stress and tension.

Caution:
- Make sure you relax and breathe.
- Keep your feet straight.

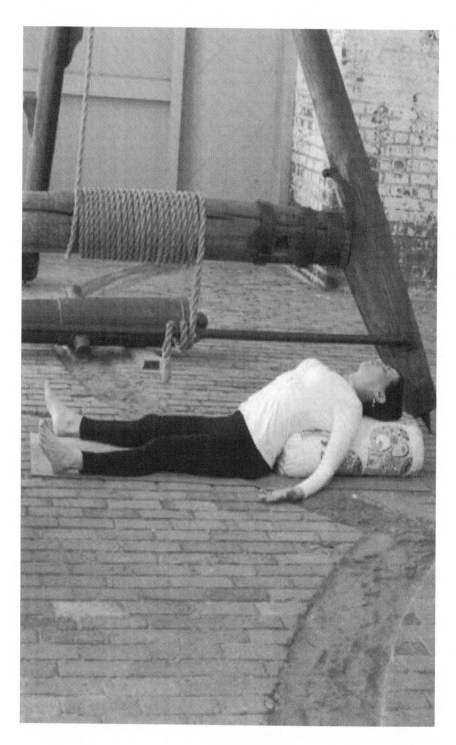

16. Supported Forward Fold Over Bolster

Directions:
- Sit on a yoga mat and place a yoga bolster in your lap.
- Tilt your tailbone backward and maintain a 30- to 35-degree curve in your lower back.
- Gently reach forward, folding your arms for a makeshift pillow and rest your forehead.
- Relax in place for five minutes.

Benefits:
- Relieves back pain.
- Restores your energy.
- Balances your nervous system.
- Relieves stress and tension.

Caution:
- Make sure you relax and breathe.
- Make sure your pelvis doesn't roll backward.
- If you have a tight lower back, elevate your hips by sitting on extra blankets so that you can enjoy a 30- to 35-degree curve in your lower back.
- You may want to add a second bolster on top of the first one, or add extra pillows or blankets for resting your forehead gently without hurting your back.

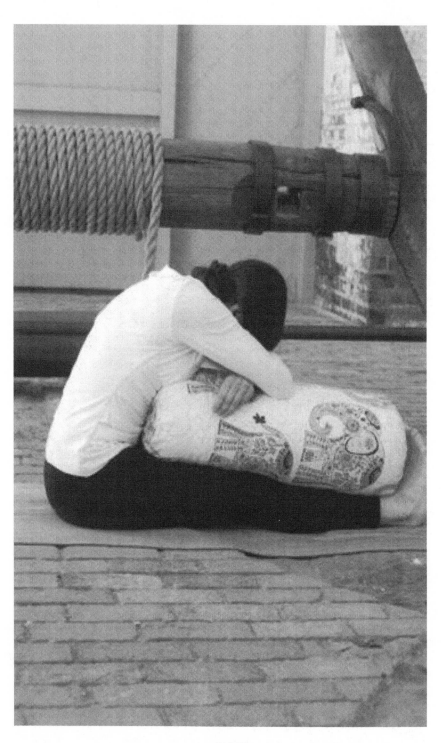

17. Child's Pose Over Bolster

Directions:
- Kneel on a yoga mat and place a yoga bolster in front of you.
- Reach forward and place your arms and hands straight ahead on the bolster.
- Sit back with your buttocks on your heels.
- Relax your head, neck and arms.
- Relax in place for five minutes.

Benefits:
- Relieves back pain.
- Restores your energy.
- Balances your nervous system.
- Relieves stress and tension.

Caution:
- Make sure you relax and breathe.
- Keep your arms as straight as possible.

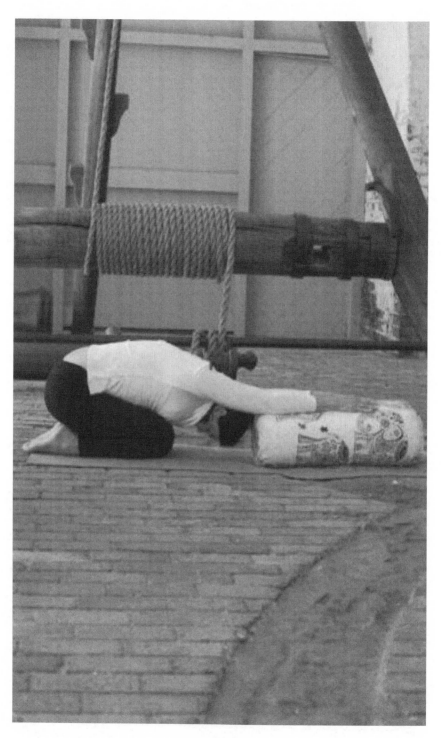

18. Supported Wide Leg Forward Bend

Directions:
- Sit on a yoga mat and place a yoga bolster in of you.
- Bring your legs as wide as you comfortably can.
- Tilt your tailbone backward and maintain a 30- to 35-degree curve in your lower back.
- Gently reach your arms forward onto the bolster.
- Relax in place for five minutes.

Benefits:
- Relieves back pain.
- Stretches your hamstrings.
- Restores your energy.
- Balances your nervous system.
- Relieves stress and tension.

Caution:
- Make sure you relax and breathe.
- Make sure your pelvis doesn't roll backward.
- If you have a tight lower back, elevate your hips by sitting on extra blankets so that you can enjoy a 30- to 35-degree curve in your lower back.
- You may want to add a second bolster on top of the first or add extra pillows or blankets to rest your forehead gently without hurting your back.

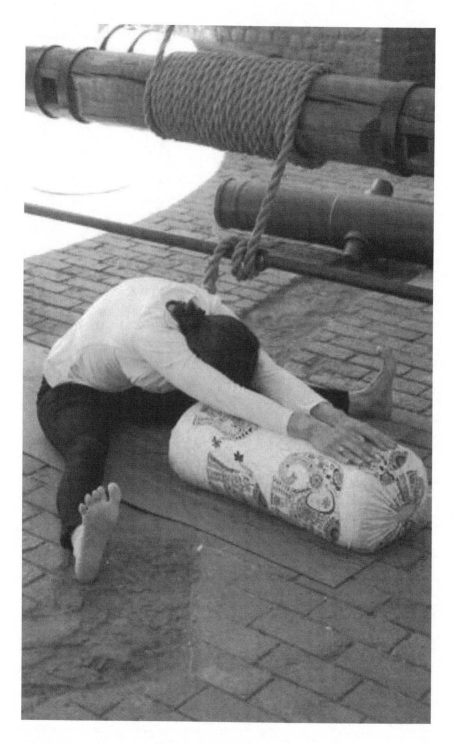

19. Reclining Butterfly Over Yoga Bolster

Directions:
- Place a yoga bolster on top of your yoga mat.
- Sit in front of your yoga bolster.
- Gently lie back with your ribs on the bolster.
- Bring the soles of your feet together.
- Support your lower legs with yoga eggs, pillows, blocks, blankets or books.
- Lengthen your arms to your sides.
- Turn your palms up to the ceiling to roll your shoulders open.
- If your neck hurts, put a pillow under your head or roll up a blanket to support your head and neck.
- Relax 5 minutes.

Benefits:
- Relieves back pain.
- Stretches your inner thighs.
- Restores your energy.
- Balances your nervous system.
- Relieves stress and tension.

Caution:
- Make sure you relax and breathe.

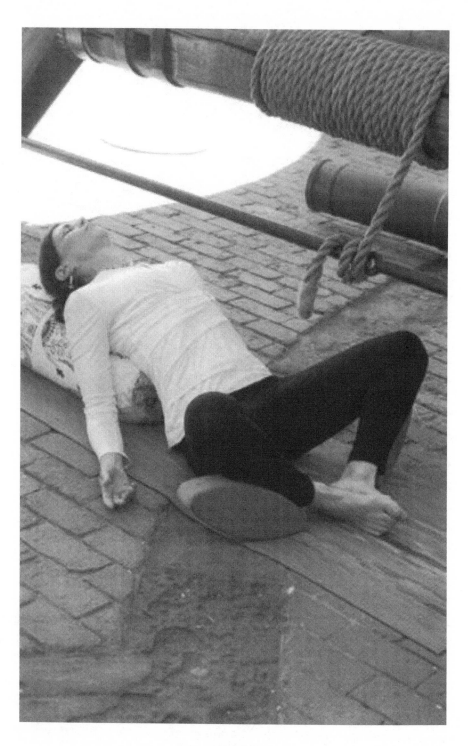

20. Wide Leg Child's Pose with Bolster

Directions:
- Kneel on a yoga mat and place a yoga bolster in front of you.
- Bring your knees comfortably apart.
- Reach forward and place your arms and hands straight ahead on the bolster.
- Sit back with your buttocks on your heels.
- Relax your head, neck and arms.
- Relax in place for five minutes.

Benefits:
- Relieves back pain.
- Restores your energy.
- Balances your nervous system.
- Relieves stress and tension.

Caution:
- Make sure you relax and breathe.
- Keep your arms as straight as possible.

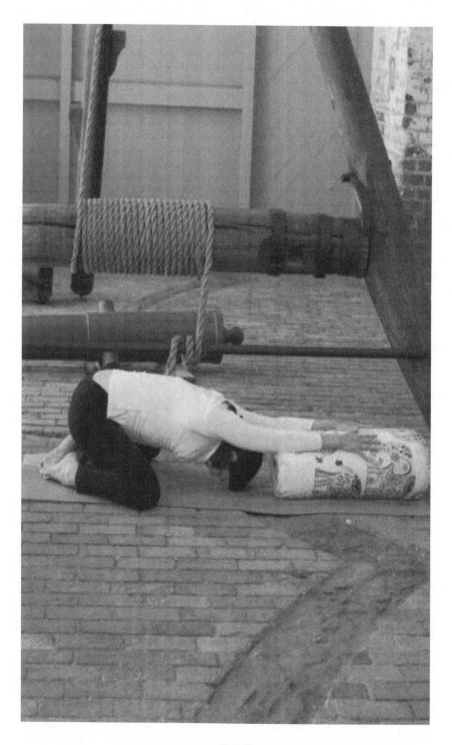

21. Reclining Twist with Yoga Bolster

Directions:
- Place a yoga bolster on the floor.
- Sit next to your bolster with your right hip on the bolster.
- Gently turn toward the bolster and fold your arms into a makeshift pillow for your forehead.
- Put your left foot on top of your right foot.
- Relax in place for five minutes.

Benefits:
- Relieves back pain.
- Restores your energy.
- Balances your nervous system.
- Releases stress and tension.

Caution:
- Make sure you relax and breathe.

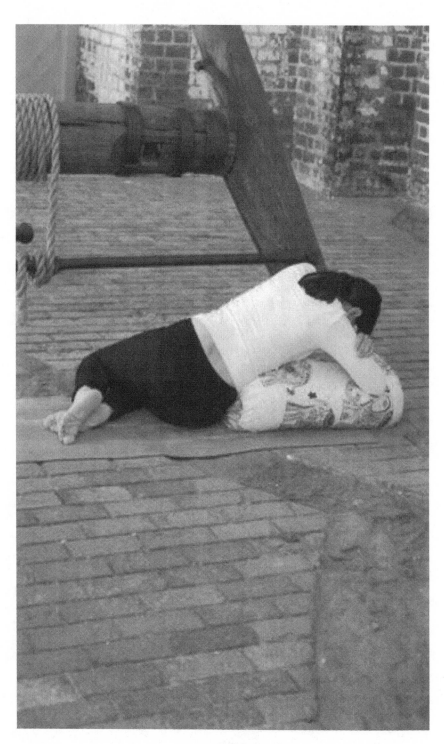

22. Supported Shoulder Stand

Directions:
- Place a yoga bolster on the floor. Ideally, you need two yoga bolsters lined up end to end, but if you don't have two bolsters, you can make do with stacks of blankets, pillows or books.
- Make a loop with your yoga strap.
- Sit on your yoga bolsters.
- Put the loop of your yoga strap around your gastrocnemius muscles (the round muscles at the top of your calf) and tighten the belt so your legs don't fall off your props.
- Lie back over the bolster with your shoulders touching the floor and your neck resting straight.
- Spread your arms at your sides with your palms turned upward.
- Relax in place for five minutes.

Benefits:
- Relieves back pain.
- Balances your thyroid gland.
- Restores your nervous system.
- Releases stress and tension.

Caution:
- Make sure you relax and breathe.
- As you come out of the pose, gently inch toward the crown of your head.

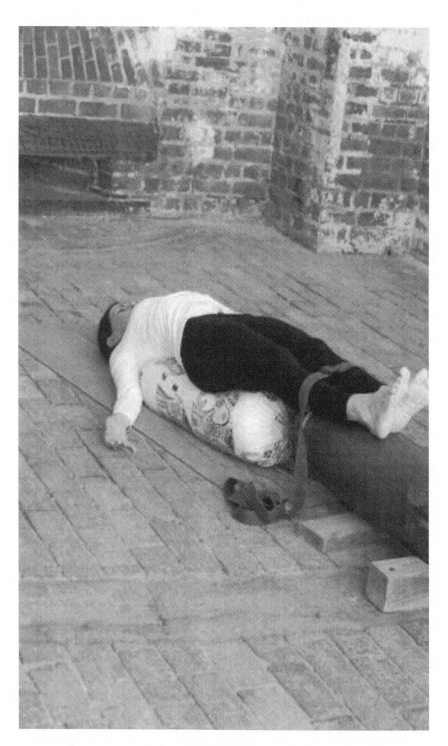

23. Legs Against the Wall Pose

Directions:
- Find a wall.
- Sit next to the wall and nestle your hips onto it.
- Swing both legs up the wall.
- Keep your legs as straight as possible.
- Drive your left heel gently into the wall.
- Draw from your left kneecap toward your left hip to accelerate the stretch in your hamstrings.
- Relax in place for five minutes.

Benefits:
- Relieves back and hip pain.
- Relaxes your spine.
- Improves your posture.
- Restores your energy.
- Clears your stress hormones and balances your nervous system.
- Gives your heart a rest.
- This is the easiest way to stretch tight hamstrings!

Caution:
- Make sure you relax and breathe.
- Keep your legs as straight as possible.

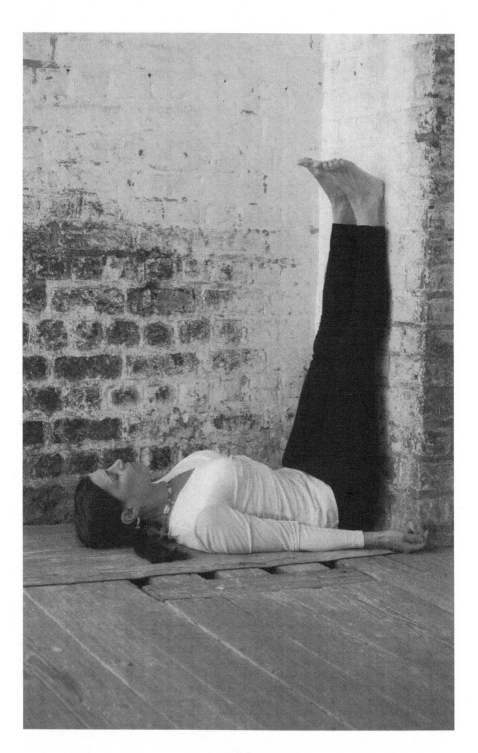

24. External Hip Rotation

Directions:
- Lie on your back, starting with both knees bent.
- Put a yoga strap on the ball of your right foot.
- Straighten your right leg as much as possible as you gently pull your right foot toward your right armpit and then swing it out to the side.
- Straighten your left leg out on the foot and be sure to point your left toes straight up to the ceiling to set the left hip bone in the socket properly.
- Keep your left hip on the floor.
- Press your left arm into the floor.
- Hold for one minute.

Benefits:
- Stretches your hip rotators.
- Relieves back and hip pain.
- Relaxes your spine.

Caution:
- Be sure to breathe deeply and relax!

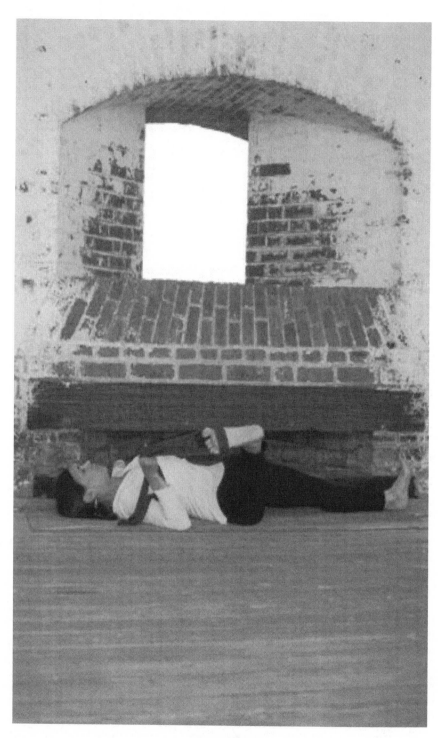

25. Four Square Hip Stretch

Directions:
- Lie on your back, starting with both knees bent.
- Put your right foot on top of your left thigh.
- Bring your right hand through the space in the middle.
- Bright your left hand behind your right thigh.
- Gently pull your bent left knee toward your chest, keeping all four corners of your hips on the ground.
- Be sure to flex your feet to accelerate the stretch in your hips.
- Hold for one minute, then repeat on the opposite side.

Benefits:
- Stretches your hips.
- Relieves back and hip pain.
- Relaxes your spine.

Caution:
- Be sure to breathe deeply and relax!
- Notice how you open your hips more deeply when you flex your feet.
- If your hips are too tight to reach with your hands, you can fold a yoga strap and thread the yoga strap behind your left knee to pull toward your chest.

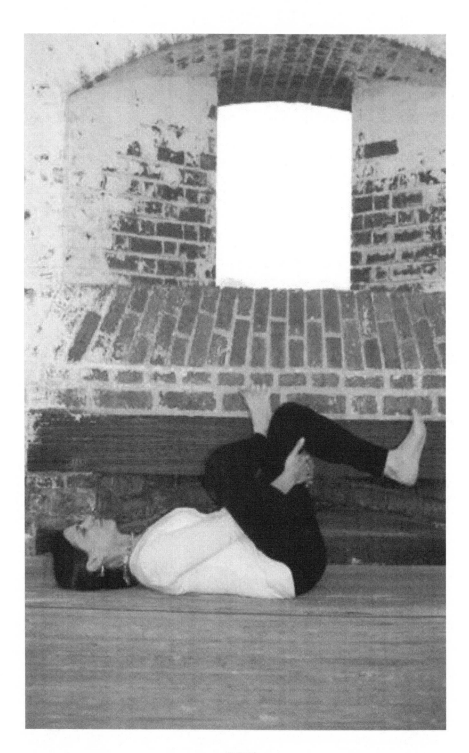

26. Fire Log Pose

Directions:
- Sit on a yoga mat with your legs straight out in front of you.
- Put your right ankle behind your left knee.
- Put a yoga egg, block, book or blanket underneath your right knee.
- Lie back.
- Put your left ankle on top of your right knee, allowing your left knee to fall open.
- Be sure to flex your feet to accelerate the stretch in your hips.
- Hold for one minute, then repeat on the opposite side.

Benefits:
- Stretches your hips.
- Relieves back and hip pain.
- Relaxes your spine.

Caution:
- Be sure to breathe deeply and relax!
- Notice how you can open your hips more deeply when you flex your feet.

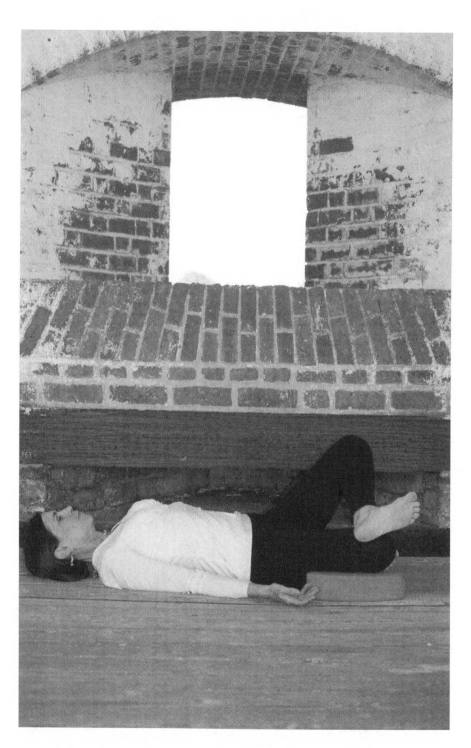

27. Prone Quadriceps Stretch

Directions:
- Make a loop with your yoga belt and put the loop around your right ankle.
- Lie face down on a yoga mat.
- Bring your knees together touching.
- Bend your right knee and grab hold of the strap.
- Pull your right heel toward your hips.
- If you are more flexible, grab hold of your right ankle and pull your heel toward your right hip.
- Hold for one minute, then repeat on the other side.

Benefits:
- Relieves hip pain.
- Stretches your quadriceps.

Caution:
- Make sure you relax and breathe.
- Make sure your knees are touching so that you stretch the four muscles of your quadriceps in alignment.

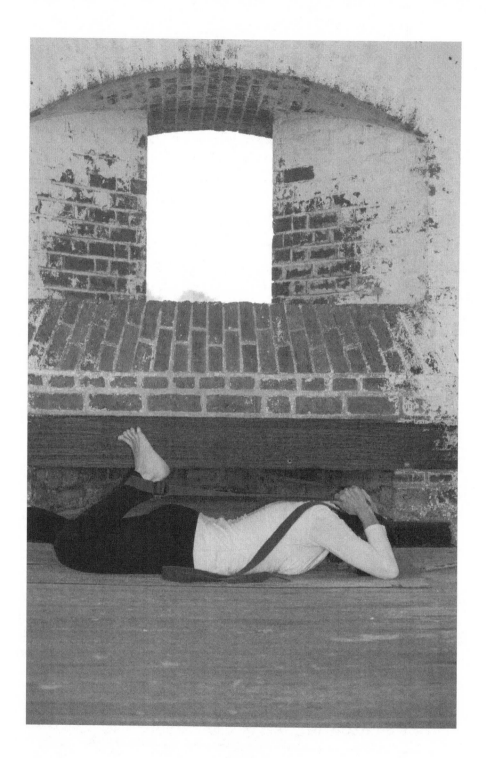

28. Double Belt Hip Traction

Directions:
- For this exercise, you need two yoga straps.
- With the first yoga strap, make a big, belted loop. To figure out how big the loop needs to be, stand up and put one end of the loop on your left foot and then guesstimate the other end of the loop as tall as your right hip.
- Now lie on the floor.
- Put one end of the loop on your left foot and straighten your left leg.
- Slide the other end of the loop into your right hip crease.
- Take the free end of your belt and tighten the loop.
- Now take the second yoga belt and put it on the ball of your right foot.
- Straighten your right leg as much as possible while you gently pull toward a 90-degree angle.
- Draw from your right kneecap toward your right hip.
- Contract your quadriceps in the front of your right thigh to increase the stretch in the hamstrings in the back of your right thigh.
- Hold one to five minutes each side.

Benefits:
- Stretches your hamstrings.
- Relieves back and hip pain.
- Relaxes your spine.
- Improves your posture.

Caution:
- Be sure to breathe deeply and relax!

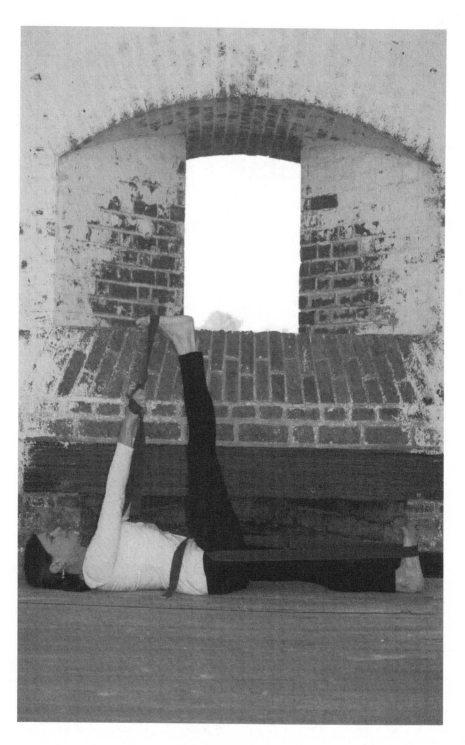

29. External Shoulder Rotation

Directions:
- Bring your right arm over your head alongside your ear.
- Wrap your shoulder. To do this, roll the inside edge out and the outside edge in.
- Lift and extend your arm a little taller.
- Bend your elbow and pat yourself on the back. You'll want to reach your hand in the direction of the opposite shoulder blade.
- Place your left hand on top of your elbow and gently depress the entire right arm. Breathe! Find the place where the stretch is interesting but not excruciating.
- Hold this stretch for at least one minute to allow your muscles, connective tissue and bones to come into gentle alignment.
- Repeat on the other side.

Benefits:
- Stretches your shoulders.
- Relaxes your spine.
- Improves your posture.

Caution:
- Be sure to breathe deeply and relax!

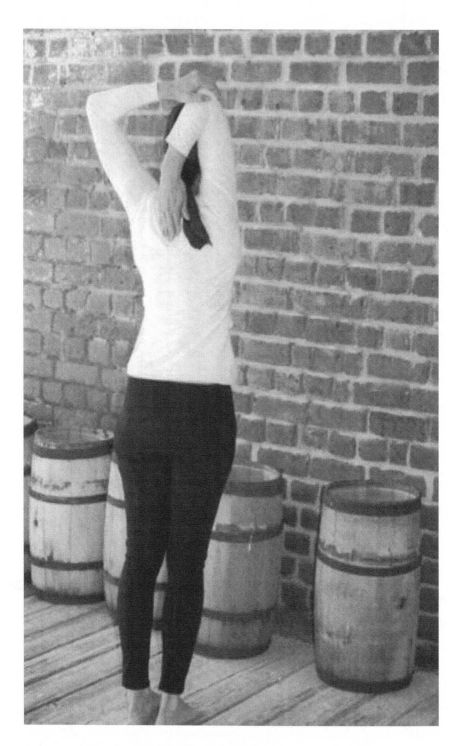

30. Internal Shoulder Rotation

Directions:

- While holding your belt, place your left hand on your lower back.
- Gently pull your left shoulder back.
- With your opposite arm, gently reach around and grab hold of your belt and pull upward. If you are super bendy, like I am simply grab hold of your left hand or fingers and tug toward your head.
- Breathe, relax and allow your body to open naturally.
- Hold this stretch for at least 60 seconds to allow your muscles, connective tissue and bones to come into gentle alignment.
- Repeat on the opposite shoulder.

Benefits:
- Stretches your shoulders.
- Relaxes your spine.
- Improves your posture.

Caution:
- Be sure to breathe deeply and relax!

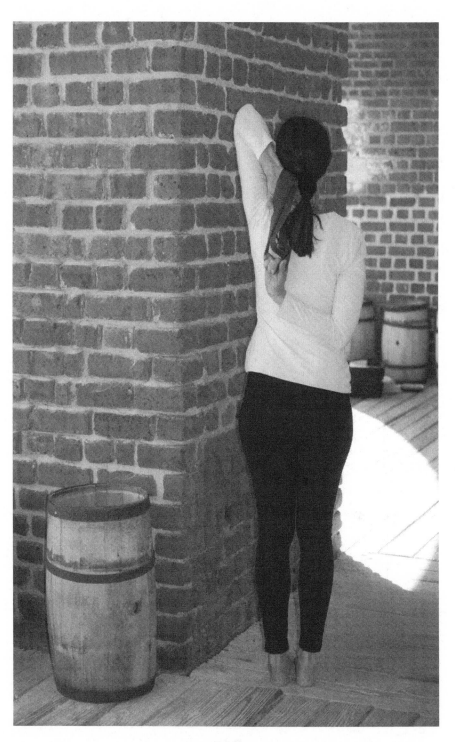

31. Shoulder Circles Lying Down

Directions:

- Lie on your right side.
- Bring your left arm over your head beside your ear with your palm facing down.
- Slowly and easily begin to move your left arm in a circle as if you were tracking the numbers on a clock.
- When you get to 6 o'clock (around your hip area), turn your palm upward.
- When you bring your arm back beside your ear, turn the palm down again.
- Continue for one minute, moving as slowly as necessary to keep the movement pain-free.
- Repeat on the opposite shoulder.

Benefits:
- Stretches your shoulders.
- Improves the range of motion in your shoulder joint.
- Relaxes your nervous system.
- Improves your posture.

Caution:
- Be sure to breathe deeply and relax!
- Keep your range of motion completely comfortable. Do not strain.

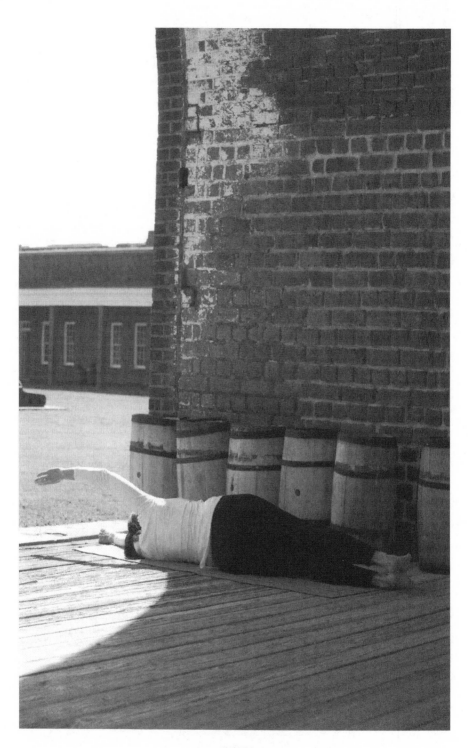

32. Eagle Arms

Directions:
- Stand or sit comfortably.
- Bend your right arm and bring it in line with your nose.
- Swing your left arm underneath your right elbow.
- Press your elbows together and bring the palms of your hands toward each another.
- Relax your upper back.
- Hold for one minute, then repeat on the opposite side.

Benefits:
- Stretches your upper back, neck and shoulders
- Relieves back, shoulder and neck pain.
- Relaxes your spine.
- Improves your posture.

Caution:
- Be sure to breathe deeply and relax!

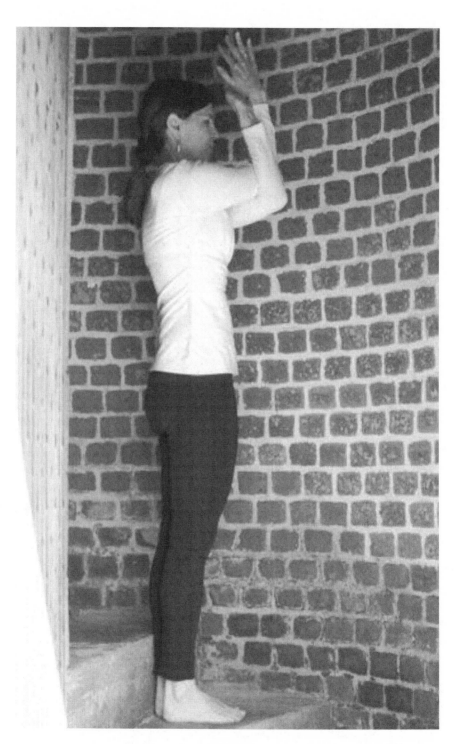

33. Tibetan Rite No. 1

Tibetan Rite No. 1

Directions:
- Stand comfortably with your arms parallel to the ground.
- Slowly and easily begin to walk your body in a clockwise circle.
- Start with one to three repetitions and work up to practicing 21 repetitions every day.

Benefits:
- Opens and balances the energy centers in your body.
- Improves your posture.
- Increases your energy level.

Caution:
- Be sure to breathe deeply and relax!
- If you get dizzy when you stop, put one hand over your navel and place the other hand on the mastoid bone behind either ear. Hold your navel and the mastoid bone until you feel a synchronized pulse. Notice how the room feels like it has stopped spinning!

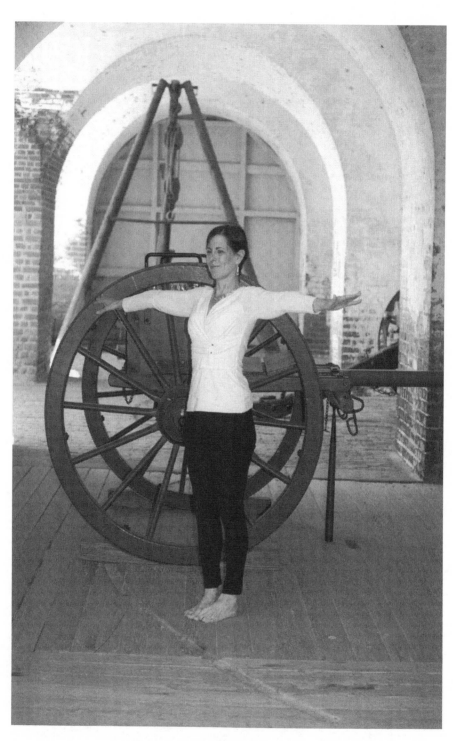

34. Tibetan Rite No. 2

Directions:
- Lie on your back on a yoga mat.
- Slide your hands under your hips to support your lower back.
- Inhale and lift your chin toward your chest.
- Exhale and pull your belly button toward your spine.
- Inhale and lift both legs toward vertical or over your head.
- Exhale and slowly lower your legs toward the floor in a controlled fashion, keeping your ankles together.
- Start with one to three repetitions and work up to practicing 21 repetitions every day.

Benefits:
- Increases your energy.
- Tones your core muscles.

Caution:
- Be sure to breathe deeply and relax!
- Do not perform this exercise if you currently suffer from back pain.
- If you have back pain, you can modify this exercise by bending your knees as you lift your legs and then again as you lower them.

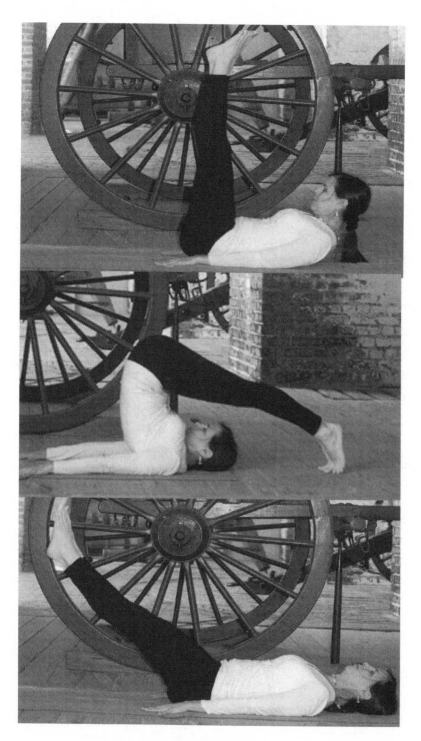

~ 353 ~

35. Tibetan Rite No. 3

Directions:
- Kneel on a yoga mat with your knees hip-width apart.
- Clasp your hands to the side of your thighs.
- Inhale and drop your chin toward your chest.
- Exhale and lengthen your neck.
- Inhale as you arch your whole body into a gentle backbend. Pull your belly button toward your spine.
- Exhale and return to the starting position.
- Start with one to three repetitions and work up to practicing 21 repetitions every day.

Benefits:
- Increases your energy.
- Tones your core muscles.

Caution:
- Be sure to breathe deeply and relax!
- If your knees feel tender, put a blanket under them for more support.

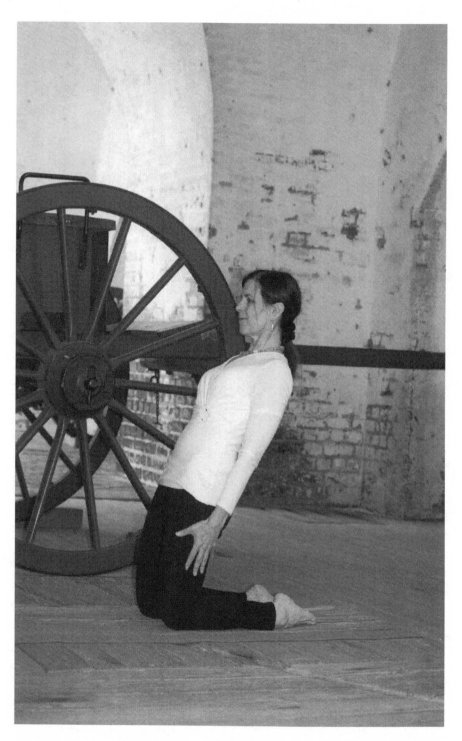

36. Tibetan Rite No. 4

Directions:
- Sit on a yoga mat with your legs straight in front of you hip-width apart.
- Inhale and drop your chin toward your chest.
- Exhale and lengthen your neck.
- Inhale as you pull your feet underneath you, pressing your hips up toward the ceiling into a tabletop position.
- Exhale and return to the starting position.
- Start with one to three repetitions and work up to practicing 21 repetitions every day.

Benefits:
- Increases your energy.
- Tones your core muscles.

Caution:
- Be sure to breathe deeply and relax!

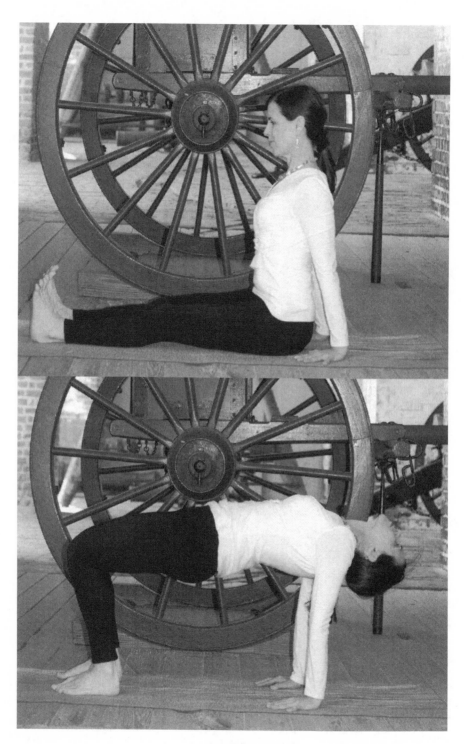

37. Tibetan Rite No. 5

Directions:
- Get down on your hands and knees on a yoga mat.
- Spread your fingers, get your wrist crease straight and lift the collarbones away from the floor as you roll the inside edge of your arms outward, wrapping your shoulders.
- Inhale and lift your hips toward the ceiling into down dog pose. Exhale and relax, holding down dog five to 10 breaths. Pull your belly button to the spine as you tilt your tailbone upward. Pull your inner thighs back.
- Now inhale and lift your heels up and come forward into extended up dog pose. Nothing should be touching the ground except your hands and feet.
- Exhale and press back to down dog pose.
- Alternate up dog pose to down dog pose.
- Start with one to three repetitions and work up to practicing 21 repetitions every day.

Benefits:
- Opens and balances your body's energy centers.
- Increases the flexibility of your spine.
- Pumps your cerebral spinal fluid.

Caution:
- Be sure to breathe deeply and relax!
- If you don't feel strong enough to alternate between up dog and down dog, just hold down dog.

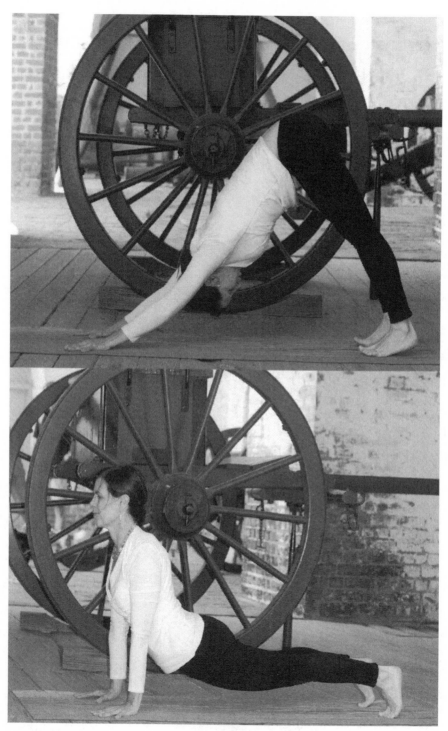

38. Traction Twist

Directions:
- Sit on a yoga mat with your knees bent and your feet as wide as your mat.
- Flex your feet.
- Drop both knees to your left.
- Get your right knee in line with your nose.
- Now lie back down on the floor.
- Press your right knee toward the ground as you pull your belly button back toward your spine.
- Hold for one minute, then repeat on the other side.

Benefits:
- Relieves back and hip pain.
- Opens your sacroiliac joint at the base of your spine.
- Relaxes your spine.
- Improves your posture.

Caution:
- Be sure to breathe deeply and relax!

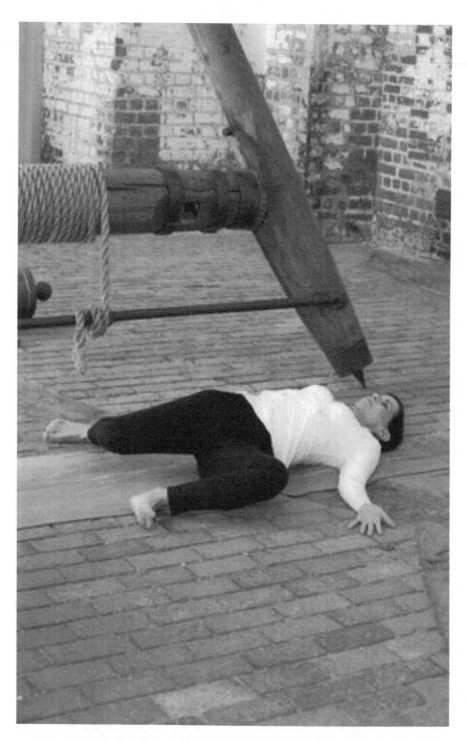

39. Mermaid

Directions:
- Sit on a yoga mat with your knees bent and your feet separated as wide as your mat.
- Flex your feet.
- Drop both knees to your left.
- Get your right knee in line with your nose.
- Press your right knee toward the ground as you pull your belly button back toward your spine.
- Now turn your body to the left, rotating each vertebra in your spine.
- Drop your chin to your chest and relax your neck.
- Hold for one minute, then repeat on the other side.

Benefits:
- Relieves back and hip pain.
- Opens your sacroiliac joint at the base of your spine.
- Increases the flexibility of your spine.
- Improves your posture.

Caution:
- Be sure to breathe deeply and relax!

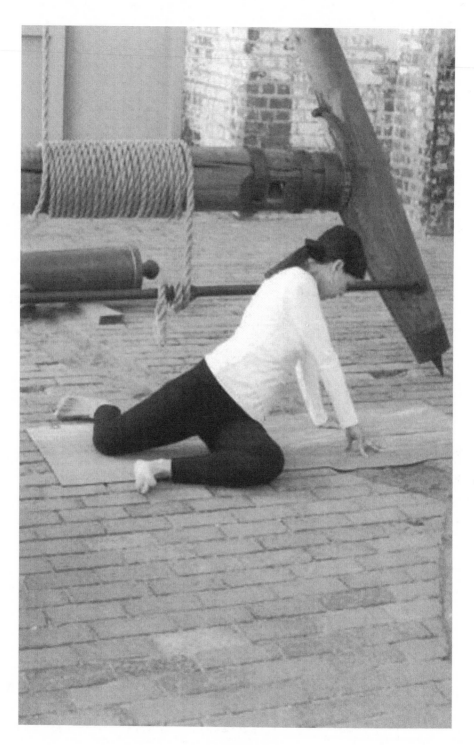

40. Scissor twist

Directions:
- Stand up straight with your right shoulder next to a wall.
- Bring your right foot in front and bring your left foot behind you with your feet three to four feet apart.
- Your front foot should be straight ahead and your back foot should be turned 45 degrees.
- Straighten both legs.
- Now bring your right arm parallel to the ground behind you as you bring your left arm in front.
- Spread your fingers and press your palms strongly into the wall to accelerate the twist.
- Keep your chin over the center of your sternum, relaxing your neck.
- Bring your front ribs forward as you rotate your back ribs behind you.
- Hold for one minute, then repeat on the other side.

Benefits:
- Relieves back pain.
- Increases the flexibility of your spine.
- Stretches your chest.
- Gently opens your hips.
- Improves your posture.

Caution:
- Be sure to breathe deeply and relax!
- Press your feet strongly into the floor.
- Keep your legs straight.

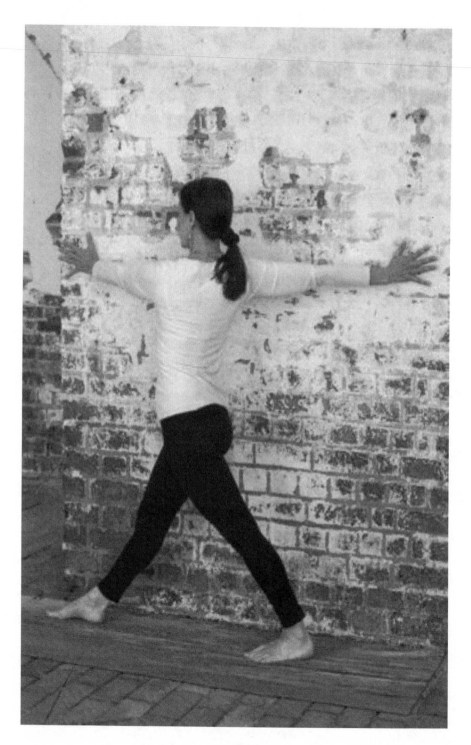

41. Foot Elevated Twist

Directions:
- Stand up straight and face a chair with your right shoulder next to a wall.
- Bring your right foot on top of the chair at roughly hip height. If necessary put a block, book, blanket or yoga egg under your foot.
- Press your left foot strongly into the floor, pulling your left inner groin back.
- Place your hands on the wall.
- Bring your front ribs forward as you rotate your back ribs behind you.
- Keep your chin over the center of your sternum, relaxing your neck.
- Hold for one minute, then repeat on the other side.

Benefits:
- Relieves back and hip pain.
- Increases the flexibility of your spine.
- Improves your posture.

Caution:
- Be sure to breathe deeply and relax!

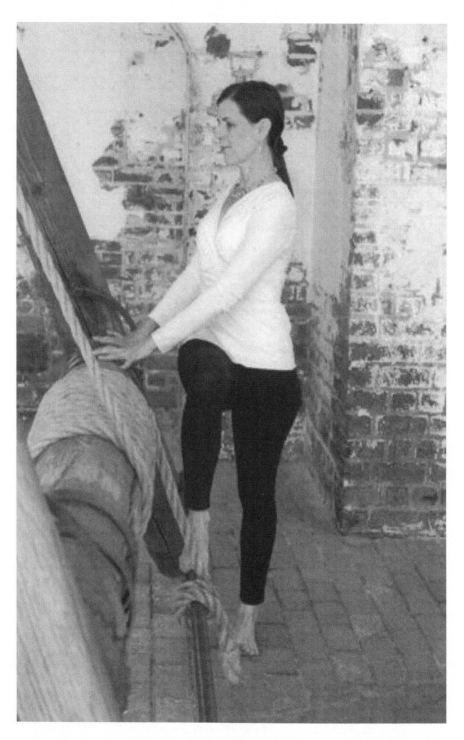

About the Photographer, Diane Fulmer

A mother of three and grandmother to seven, Diane Fulmer discovered her passion for photography after retiring from her career in nursing.

You can see more of her excellent work at www.dianebookerphotography.com.

"My hope is that my photographs will evoke some emotion and a wish to linger," Diane says.

Diane Fulmer returned to Armstrong Atlantic State University in Savannah to learn the deeper aspects of image making, with a strong love for printing from the negative in a digital world. Diane immersed herself in classical black and white and lith printing, a darkroom process used widely in Europe. She continues to explore new techniques including the art of digital photography.

Although Diane prefers coastal scenes, she also enjoys architecture, still life and portraits captured in the landscape. She strives to bring emotion and meaning to her photographs and uses SLR and medium format film and digital cameras.

Her nursing background and desire to share her passion led her to volunteer at Hospice Savannah as photographer for End of Life Family Photographer, a program she started in 2007.

Diane continues to develop her darkroom skills through independent studies at AASU and demonstrates her Lith and Sepia techniques for Photography classes at AASU under Linda Jensen, Professor of Photography. In March 2010 she attended a seven-day workshop with John Sexton in Carmel, California to refine her photography and darkroom skills.

About The Author, Catherine Carrigan

Catherine Carrigan is a medical intuitive healer and Amazon No. 1 bestselling author. She has taught yoga for 21 years and empowers her clients to alleviate pain and suffering through a wide range of natural healing methods.

You can connect with her on Facebook at
https://www.facebook.com/catherinecarriganauthor
Follow her on Twitter at https://twitter.com/CSCarrigan
Read her blog at www.catherinecarrigan.com
Check out her websites at **www.catherinecarrigan.com**
and www.unlimitedenergynow.com
Connect with her on LinkedIn at:
www.linkedin.com/in/catherinecarrigan/
Keep up with news about her books at:
https://www.goodreads.com/author/show/638831.Catherine_Carrigan
Sign up for her newsletter at: http://bit.ly/1C4CFOC

You can read testimonials from her clients here:
http://catherinecarrigan.com/testimonials/

Training in Fitness

- Certified Personal Fitness Trainer: A.C.E. certified in Personal Fitness Training
- Corrective High-Performance Exercise Kinesiologist (C.H.E.K) Practitioner, Level I: C.H.E.K. Institute.
- Certified Group Exercise Instructor: A.C.E. certified in Group Exercise
- A.C.E. Specialty Recognitions: Strength Training and Mind-Body Fitness
- Exercise Coach, C.H.E.K. Institute
- Certified Yoga Teacher: 500-hour Yoga Teacher through Lighten Up Yoga; six 200-hour certifications through Integrative Yoga Therapy, the White Lotus Foundation, and the Atlanta Yoga Fellowship, Lighten Up Yoga and Erich Schiffmann teacher training (twice)
- Practitioner of qi gong, Chinese martial arts
- Certified Older Adult Fitness Trainer through the American Institute of Fitness Educators

Training in Nutrition

- Food Healing Level II Facilitator
- Holistic Lifestyle Coach though the C.H.E.K. Institute, Level 3

- Certified Sports Nutritionist through the American Aerobics Association International/International Sports Medicine Association
- Author, *Healing Depression: A Holistic Guide* (New York: Marlowe and Co., 1999), a book discussing nutrition and lifestyle to heal depression without drugs
- Schwarzbein Practitioner though Dr. Diana Schwarzbein, an expert in balancing hormones naturally

Training in Healing

- Specialized Kinesiology and Life Coaching through Sue Maes of London, Ontario, Canada
- Self-Empowerment Technology Practitioner
- Brain Gym, Vision Circles and Brain Organization instructor through the Educational Kinesiology Foundation
- Certified Touch for Health Practitioner
- Thai Yoga Body Therapy
- Flower Essence Practitioner
- Reiki Master, Usui Tradition
- Life Coaching through Sue Maes' Mastering Your Knowledge Mentorship Program and Peak Potentials
- Medical Intuitive Readings and Quantum Healing

Other Training

- Health and fitness columnist
- Playwright of 12 plays, including three produced in New York City
- Past spokesperson for the Depression Wellness Network
- Phi Beta Kappa graduate of Brown University
- Former national spokesperson for Johnson & Johnson
- Owner and co-host, Total Fitness Radio Show
- Author of the Amazon No. 1 best seller *What Is Healing? Awaken Your Intuitive Power for Health and Happiness*
- Author of the Amazon No. 1 best seller, *Unlimited Energy Now*
- Author of the Amazon No. 1 best seller, *Banish the Blues Now*
- Author of *What Is Social Media Today? Get Ready to Win the Game of Social Media*
- Author of the Amazon No. 1 best seller, *What Is Social Media Today? Hashtags, Keywords and You, Oh My!*

About the Cover Design

This photograph of two buckeye butterflies was taken at Greenleaf Gardens in South Carolina by the author Catherine Carrigan.

Butterflies symbolize personal transformation, playfulness and elevation of your soul. May this book empower you to transform your pain and suffering into lightness of being, joy and delight.

Cover design by Ramajon Cogan

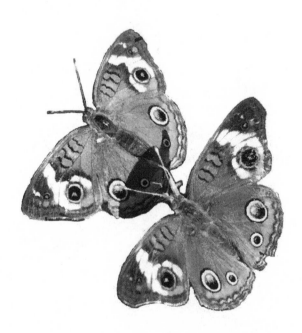

Acknowledgements

I'd like to thank the great team that made this book possible.

Thanks to Tony Kessler who went above and beyond the call of duty to edit this book.

Thanks to Diane Fulmer who took amazing yoga photos and left her mark on this book by sharing with us her artistic style.

Thanks to RamaJon who formatted the interior and the cover and who helped make this book my best work to date.

And last, but by no means least, Dixie, my constant companion and muse.

What is

HEALING?

Awaken Your Intuitive Power for Health and Happiness

CATHERINE CARRIGAN

About *What Is Healing? Awaken Your Intuitive Power for Health and Happiness*

In this book, you will:

- Learn how unconditional love can awaken your intuitive gifts.
- Reveal how to open your heart to access your highest intelligence.
- Uncover how to communicate with your angels and spiritual guides.
- Awaken your own psychic abilities.
- Identify the key aspects of a medical intuitive reading.
- Discern how addiction to staying sick can keep you from healing.
- Reveal the blessing behind a mental or physical breakdown.
- Grasp the four key difficulties that lead to health problems.
- Empower your own spiritual growth.

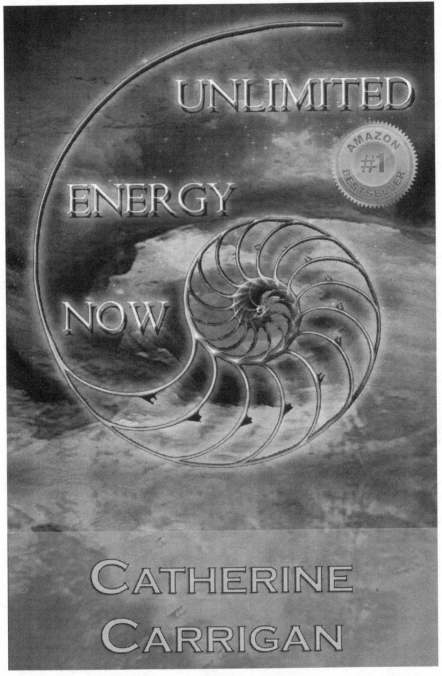

UNLIMITED ENERGY NOW

AMAZON #1 BESTSELLER

CATHERINE CARRIGAN

About *Unlimited Energy Now*

Discover the secrets of how you can experience unlimited energy *now:*

- Learn how to operate your body at its very best.
- Master your own energy system.
- Resolve the emotions that drain you.
- Connect to your highest intelligence.
- Inspire yourself to connect more deeply to your infinite, eternal and unwavering support from your soul.

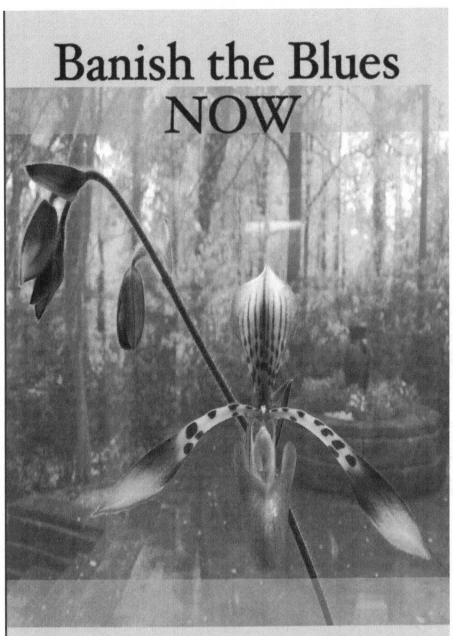

Banish the Blues
NOW

Catherine Carrigan

Banish the Blues NOW addresses:

HEALING DEPRESSION WITHOUT DRUGS using NATURAL HEALING remedies. Did you know that the Centers for Disease Control and Prevention reports that **11 percent of all Americans over the age of 12 take antidepressants**?

Women are more likely than men to take these drugs at every level of severity of depression.
Non-Hispanic white persons are more likely to take antidepressants than are non-Hispanic black and Mexican-American persons.
Of those **taking antidepressants, 60 percent have taken them for more than 2 years, and 14 percent have taken the drugs for more than 10 years.** About 8 percent of persons aged 12 and over with no current depressive symptoms took antidepressant medication.

Despite the widespread acceptance of natural healing methods, from 1988-1994 through 2005-2008, the rate of antidepressant use in the United States among all ages increased nearly 400 percent.

It is my prayer that my new book will be of service in teaching you how to heal depression without drugs, banishing your blues FOR GOOD!

FOREWARD By Abram Hoffer, M.D., Ph.D., FRCP(C) Editor, *The Journal of Orthomolecular Medicine*

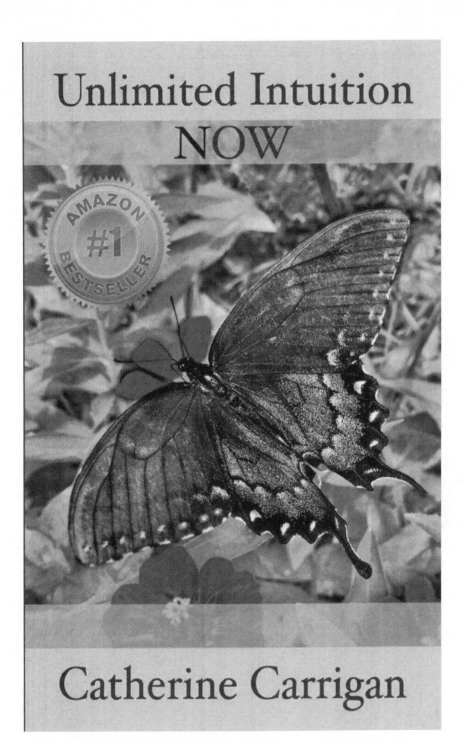

Unlimited Intuition NOW

Catherine Carrigan

AMAZON #1 BESTSELLER

READ *UNLIMITEDINTUITION NOW*
TO DEVELOP YOUR OWN PSYCHIC ABILITIES SO
THAT YOU CAN RECEIVE GUIDANCE FROM YOUR
SOUL.

How you will benefit:

- Pray to open your soul guidance.
- Learn how to read the energy in your. chakras with a pendulum
- Tune in to read your own body.
- Discover how to read the body of another person.
- Discern how much life force is in your food.
- Focus to tell if food is really good for your body.
- Practice how to muscle test yourself.
- Raise your vibration to listen to your angels.
- Get your ego out of the way so you can listen to divine guidance.
- Stay connected with loved ones when you are apart.
- Open your psychic centers of clairaudience, claircognizance, clairsentience and clairvoyance.
- Avoid other people's ego projections to see what's really going on.
- Protect your energy so you feel safe and grounded at all times and in all places.
- Stay out of trouble in dangerous situations.
- Understand how your different psychic gifts actually work.
- Deepen your connection to God and feel supported on all level

What is Social Media
TODAY

Get Ready to Win

The Game of Social Media

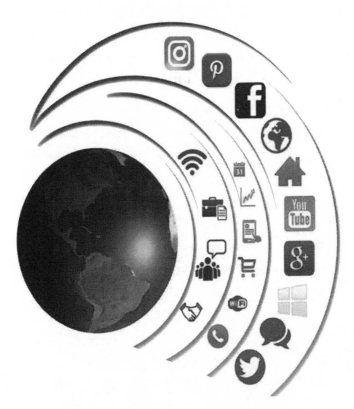

Catherine Carrigan

What is Social Media Today
Where Social Media is Fun

Lose your fear of social media

Tackle Twitter

Make friends with Facebook

Become a Youtube superstar

Create compelling viral content

Grow and brand your business

Hit page one of Google

Build your audience

Increase your income

Develop raving fans

What is
Social Media Today

Hashtags, Keywords And You
Oh My!

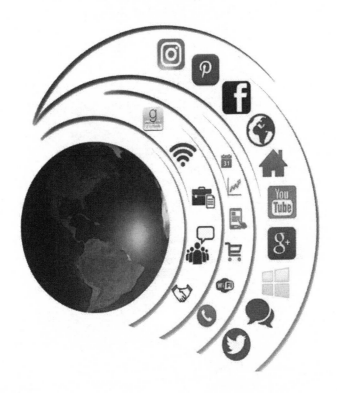

Catherine Carrigan

Are you making mistakes that keep you broke, without customers, readers or the success you deserve?

Keywords and Hashtags are the foundation for successful social media marketing.

What is Social Media Today is a broad based social media marketing training program.

You will have a consistent social media presence and will be posting like an expert in no time.

Read this book to learn how to use keywords and hashtags to build your tribe online and draw more customers for your products, books, services and business.

Made in the USA
Lexington, KY
28 August 2017